Dear John.

Best Wishes for a
fine birthday.

x/0

grey

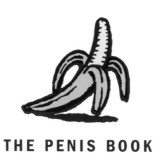

THE PENIS BOOK

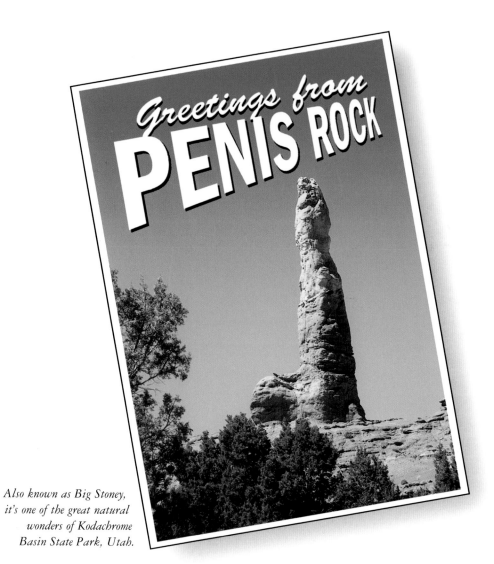

Greetings from **PENIS ROCK**

Also known as Big Stoney, it's one of the great natural wonders of Kodachrome Basin State Park, Utah.

THE PENIS BOOK

Joseph Cohen

BROADWAY

For Bob.
Who inspires me with
laughter, wisdom and love.

Published by Broadway Books
a division of Random House

Produced by Fresh Ideas Daily
New York City

Designed by SimonGraphics.com
New York City

Library of Congress Cataloging–in–Publication Data
Cohen, Joseph
The Penis Book / Joseph Cohen.
p.cm.
1. Penis—Humor.   I. Title.
PN6231.P344/C64 2004
818'.5402—dc22   2003069613

ISBN: 0-7679-1753-7
©2004 Joseph Cohen
©2004 Broadway Books, a division of Random House

Previous Design by Tom Dolle Design, New York City

Printed in Singapore

10 9 8 7 6 5 4 3 2

You have one.

You want one.

You love them.

You hate them...

The penis.

It's hard to imagine
that something tinier
than a chihuahua
can stir up so many
emotions,
escapades,
steamy page-turners,
phone sex businesses,
visits to the shrink,
babies,
dirty jokes,
sleepless nights,
dreamy sighs,
lies,
embarrassed giggles.

And so much fun.

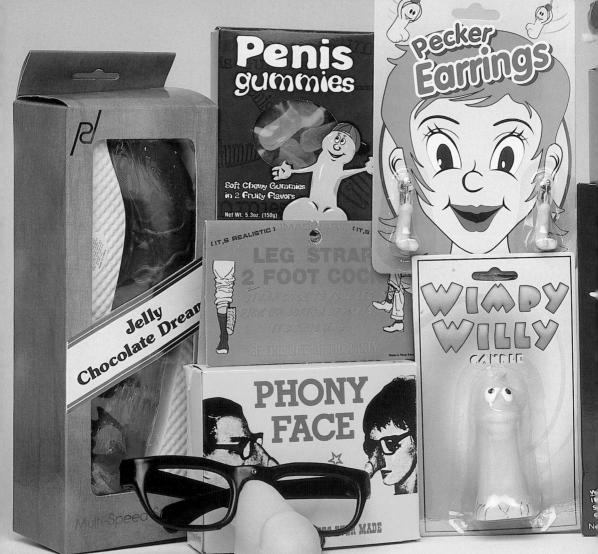

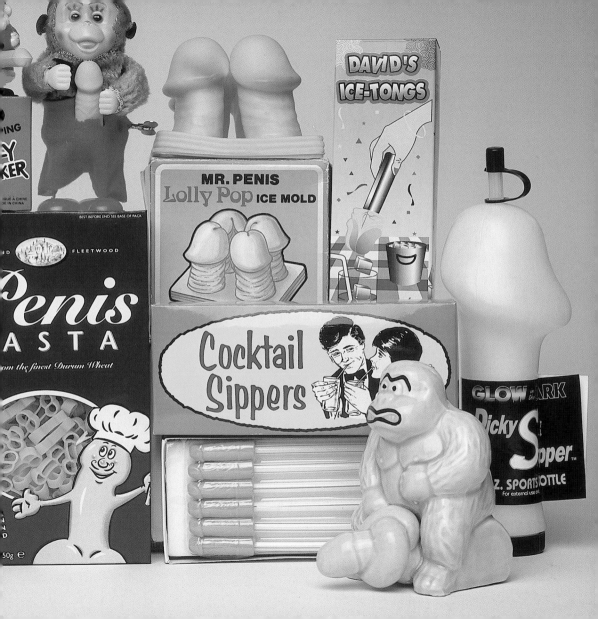

Step right up

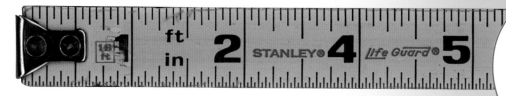

Most guys dream of sporting a long, thick porno porker instead of their trusty cocktail frank. Forget it. If you're like most men, no yardstick is necessary for this assignment. While there are some amazing exceptions to the ruler, here's the law of averages: **The average length of a flaccid penis is 3.9 inches, with a girth of 3.7 inches. The average length of an erect penis is 5.9 inches, with a girth of 4.9 inches. Penises usually reach their manly max by the time a male turns 17.**

SWEET REVENGE. The shorter a guy's penis, the bigger it blossoms. Many chaps whose members are in the three-inch range when flaccid can look forward to organs that double in size when fully erect. Their hunkier buddies, on the other hand, almost never experience such generous growth... although they're still ahead of the game.

BIG NOSE, BIG HOSE? Not necessarily. While we've all heard tales about beefy hands, noses and earlobes being surefire signs that a huge dick is waiting in the wings, thou-

drop your pants.

MADE IN U.S.A. 10 APP'D 339 TC 11 14 15

sands of measurements over the years show no correlation. Penis size is very much a product of heredity and genetics, not the size of your loafers.

THE INCREDIBLE SHRINKING DICK.
Fear, stress and icy ocean water will all shrink a penis down to grade-school dimensions. During annual physical exams, approximately one-third of all males will feel a need to explain their diminished equipment, uttering something like: "Doc, it's really a lot bigger when I get out of here."

BLOW OFF THE DUST AND USE IT.
It's incredibly beneficial to keep your pecker sexually (and safely) active, most urologists agree. Erections fill your penis with oxygen-rich blood, essential for the survival of the smooth muscle tissue within the arteries of your ding-dong. A shortage of oxygen will eventually lead to a build-up of collagen, making erections a sweet memory. So use that tool!

ENLARGEMENT SURGERY? Don't be ridiculous. Phalloplasty can lead to scarring, erection discomforts and impotence. Love your weenie the way it is. And lose some weight.

The Queer Penis

Oh the stories these frisky sauçisson could tell. *Homo-erectus-as-often-as-possible* is a life force all its own, eagerly squirming its way above the waistband of basket-enhancing $2^{(x)}$ist underwear to sniff out the action. The queer penis is a precocious pickle...swordfighting with other inquisitive peckers at the age of 12, circle-jerking just a few pimples later, swelling in a dormitory mate's mouth by 18 and, ultimately, discovering the penetrating world of lovemaking that begins with another's male's tender/torrid kiss.

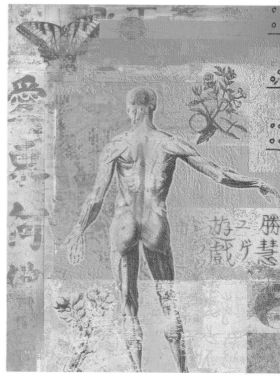

The most upbeat news from the world of queer dicks is that they're ready to settle down. After years of operating on cruise control, countless homo cockowners are shifting lanes for that happy destination called commitment. What a change. What a cozy, serene time it is for road-weary penises as they nap during *Antiques Roadshow* and expand just a tad in front of the Makita drill display at Home Depot. The queer penis is finding its home at last. ■

The Straight Penis

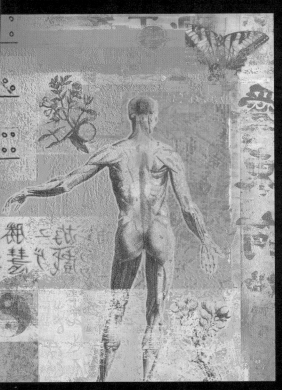

Ah, the lure of eager labial folds, welcoming the hung hetero in their moist embrace. From the days of testosterone-driven youth, the straight penis hungers for shelter. It can be the downy *frottage* of a pillow from L.L.Bean. A juicy blowjob with its Maybelline Pinkissimo smooch. Or, later, the finesse of an artful *shtup* with a serious girlfriend, where the manly rod—no longer in a rush—is serenaded by quivering moans of female pleasure. And try to find an adventurous pecker that hasn't attempted a house call at a lady's back door.

A born comparison shopper, the hetero hose is forever checking out the equipment of other guys at the gym (and guessing which ones were just plumped up at the plastic surgeon's office). Even the straightest suburban dicks are borrowing a few grooming tips from their queer brethren, sporting the streamlined profile of shaved balls and pubic hair that's groomed to the max. It's a tempting new package. "I'm an object of desire!" it seems to say. ∎

THE AVERAGE MALE...

between the ages of 15 and 60
will ejaculate 30 to 50 quarts of semen
containing 350 to 500 billion sperm cells.

Average volume of ejaculate:	*0.5 to 1 teaspoon*
Chief ingredient:	*fructose*
Caloric content:	*5 calories per teaspoon*
Protein content:	*6 milligrams per teaspoon*
Average number of ejaculatory spurts:	*3 to 10*
Average speed of ejaculation:	*25 miles per hour*
Average interval of ejaculatory contractions:	*0.8 seconds*
Average duration of orgasm:	*4 seconds*
Farthest medically recorded ejaculation:	*27.5 inches*
Average number of sperm cells in ejaculate of a healthy man:	*200 to 600 million*
Average number in ejaculate of an infertile man:	*50 million*
Average swimming speed:	*1 to 4 millimeters per minute*

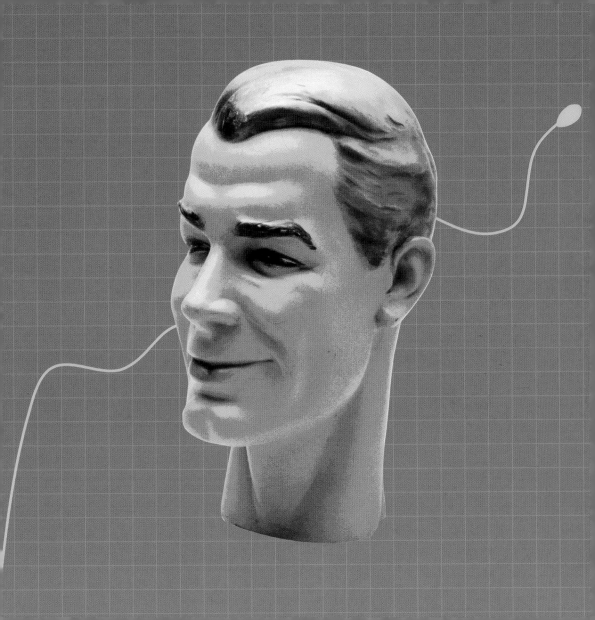

Actually, testicles are about 4˚F cooler than the rest of a man's body temperature, providing the ideal climate for copious sperm production. (Avoid hot tubs and tight bikini underwear if you're trying to conceive.) ✳ About 90 percent of the male hormone testosterone originates in the testicles before it enters the bloodstream and travels throughout the body. ✳ European testicles tend to weigh about twice as much as their Chinese cousins. ✳ To prevent a life-long collision course, the left testicle hangs lower in about 85% of the male population and is usually a bit larger. ✳ When taking an oath, our biblical ancestors would place their hands over the testicles of a witness to indicate their sincerity and honesty. Words like "testify" and "testament" all derive from this unique association. ✳ Recent studies from England indicate that guys with large testicles had sex about 30% more often than their smaller-balled brothers and were more likely to cheat on their partners. ✳ Eunuchs of the Chinese Imperial Court often carried their pickled testicles in jars which they displayed around their necks. ✳ Testicular cancer has the highest cure rate of any cancer when it is detected in its early stage. Monthly self-exams are encouraged and should take place after a shower when the scrotal skin is relaxed.✳

While testicles deserve tender loving care, men also love having their balls

Great Balls Of

squeezed, sucked, slapped and tugged. He'll let you know when you're going too far. ✳ Each September, Montana's Original Testicle Festival serves more than 4,500 pounds of deep-fried bull's testicles, better known as Mountain Oysters. No bones. Dig right in. ✳ Vary your vocabulary for a rich conversation: Family Jewels, Nuts, Clangers, Spunk Holders, Jizz Sack, Cojones, Plums, Kiwis, Hairy Prunes, Fuzz Balls, Sweat Sack, Poucheroo, Tea Bags, Mike & Mo and the Melon Boys are all lively substitutes.

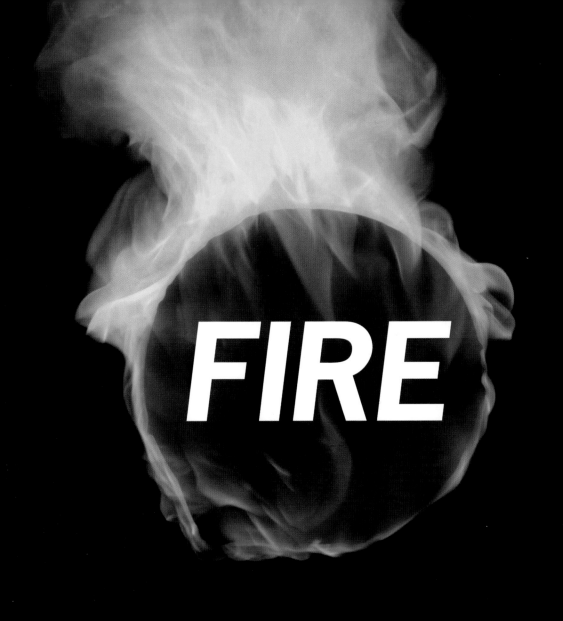

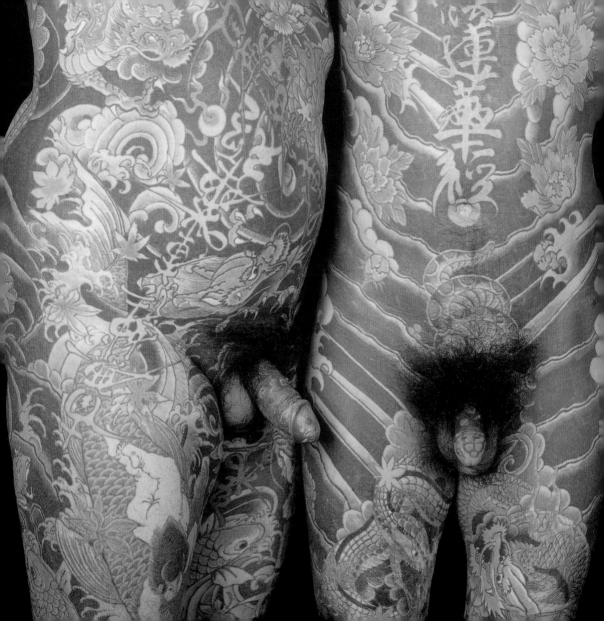

Taboo

They're called *Irezumi*, a rather secretive group of Japanese men and women, often drawn from the underworld, who transform their bodies into living works of art. The penis is the last part of the anatomy to be tattooed and it's always the most painful procedure, with the tattoo master focusing on a tiny section per session.

Even after death, these adorned bodies continue to amaze. Some 300 half-body and full-body skins have been preserved in airtight frames and sold to museums and private collectors. Interested? A few years ago, a half-body tattoo was auctioned for $50,000.

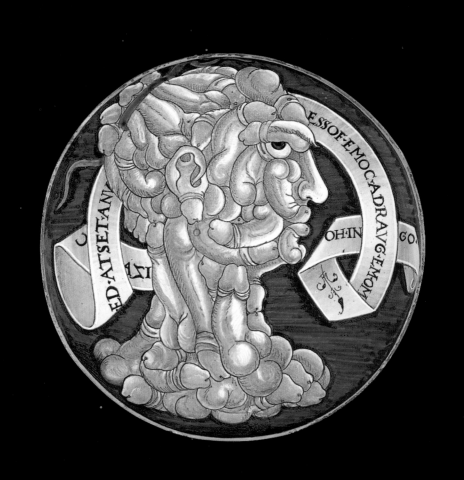

Who are you calling a Dickhead?

The venerable Ashmolean Museum of Art and Archaeology at the University of Oxford is a stodgy grande dame on the outside. But inside, she's high-kicking with saucy glee since purchasing one of the bawdiest and rarest maiolica plates of the 16th century for a whopping $360,000.

Painted by Francesco Urbino in 1536, this Renaissance wonder is a parody of the charming bella-donna style of dishes, which showcased the portraits of virtuous young girls. On the banderole, reading right to left and written in reverse, is the inscription *"Ogni homo me guarda come fosse una testa de cazi"*…translated: "Every man looks at me as if I were a head of dicks."

Look carefully, and you'll count at least 34 penises, including a pierced member by her right ear. Clearly a lass with a lot more on her mind than rushing home to cook the lasagna, she's the stiffest competition the Mona Lisa has seen in years.

You're not alone

Estimates hover around 152 million men worldwide experiencing problems with their erectile choreography. With nine out of ten men not yet seeking treatment, analysts predict the erectile dysfunction market will rise to almost $5 billion by 2006.

Moan / groan

■ A Viagra truck was hijacked. The police are looking for two hardened criminals. They expect a stiff sentence under the penal code.
■ Hear about the guy who overdosed with his E.D. pills? The funeral home couldn't close the coffin for three days.

Like wow

Say goodbye to flaccid flora. An Israeli scientist discovered that by adding Viagra to containers filled with cut blooms, the flowers stayed fresh and erect for a week longer than usual thanks to an increased supply of nitric oxide.

Happy to report

Open discussion about ED is encouraging more and more men to visit their doctor for a regular check-up as well as for that Rx of bountiful promise. Just as encouraging, Viagra & Pals is shrinking the demand for useless aphrodisiacs made from the penises of tigers, rhinos, elephants and many other macho, endangered species.

How they work

All of these drugs inhibit the enzyme PDE-5, thus relaxing and widening the muscles in the arterial wall of the penis and allowing more blood to flow through. The penis grows and becomes erect. Meanwhile, the veins that carry blood away from the penis get compressed, making the member larger. No matter how clever the pill, you've got to be sexually stimulated. It all starts in the head between a guy's ears.

COMING RIGHT UP!

Long, long ago, in the dark ages of 1998, a little blue pill called Viagra kicked erectile dysfunction out of the bedroom and onto center stage. Unimaginable conversations like, "Hey, you go limp? Me, too!" became almost cool, now that a dependable woody was as close as a 45-minute countdown.

More than one billion V's have been sold worldwide to more than 20 million men. Viagra picked up a Nobel Prize the year it was introduced. And it poked its way into the venerable Oxford English Language Dictionary. But the last word on ED wonder drugs is still being written. The competition is hotter than a hard-on. Levitra (a perky shade of orange) seems to kick in quicker and mixes well with food. While the eager beavers behind Cialis (yellow, fellow) are boasting a whole weekend of bliss, with sexual prowess lasting up to 36 hours. Confidence never felt so good.

4 COCKS
4 COCKBURNs
11 DICKMANs

12 WOODYs
1 ROD
3 SALAMIs

4 PECKERs
1 PECKERMAN
29 DICKs

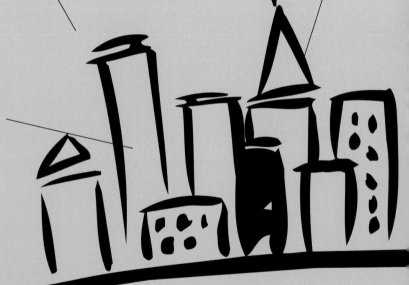

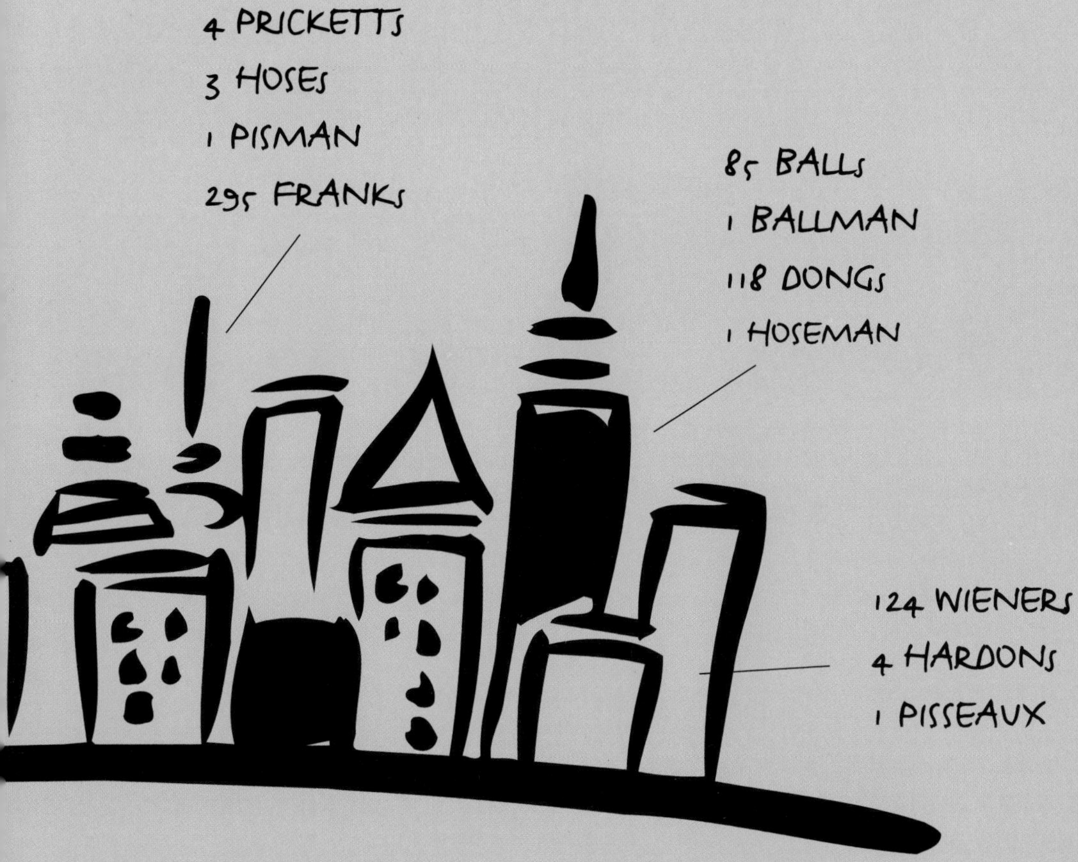

4 PRICKETTS
3 HOSES
1 PISMAN
295 FRANKS

85 BALLS
1 BALLMAN
118 DONGS
1 HOSEMAN

124 WIENERS
4 HARDONS
1 PISSEAUX

CockTalk

What Guys Really Think About Their Most Precious Possession

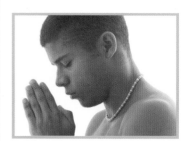

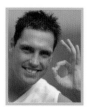

LANDON

Penis name:
Perky

Best qualities:
People tell me my dick has a lot of personality. That's because it always has this happy semi-erect look…like it wants to talk to you.

Fantasy time:
Perky could definitely use some extra girth. I'd like it to be more of a handful when I grab it, like a Sicilian dockworker's, even though I'm Jewish.

My penis says:
"I'm tired of all those smelly dark holes. I want to vacation under the sun and do nothing!"

Erect size: 6 inches

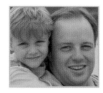

ALAN

Penis name:
Lollypop

Profile:
My little boy thinks I have the biggest penis in the whole world and can't wait for his to be like mine. My wife thinks my pecker is adorable, but she wishes I'd do something with it. She's pretty frustrated.

The truth:
I'm always tired. I don't even masturbate anymore when I'm on a business trip. I used to have so much fun with my dick. Now it's just pee and shake.

Voice of the penis:
"I'm sick of your screaming kids. You and the missus need to get away…or else!"

Erect size: 6.5 inches

EDUARDO

Penis names: El Humongo and Sea Monster

Thumbs up:
Thank you Virgin Mother for blessing me with a really big pene. Some women get kinda scared when they see it…but once they get on top of me, they're squealing like they're on a ride at Great Adventure.

Room for improvement:
My dick gets this weird purple color when I'm all excited. It looks like it's choking.

Tales from my tool:
"You don't use condoms enough. Jerkhead, do you want to end up like your cousin Felix?"

Erect size: 8.75 inches

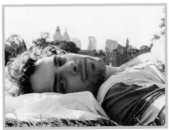

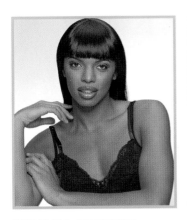

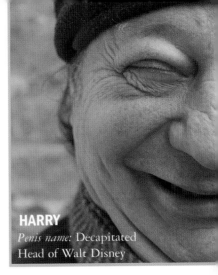

MICKEY
Penis name: Michelangelo

Strong points:
My dick is incredibly smooth and it has this beautiful even color. People tell me it looks like a sculpture, but it's warm and you can touch it as much as you want.

Wish list:
I'd love two more inches, because nothing turns me on more than watching my dick go in and out. Goodbye…hello again.

If it could talk:
"Stop taking me for granted. Pat me dry instead of rubbing me with a cheap towel. Don't get upset when I don't cum."

Erect size: 6 inches

FANTASIA (REUBEN)
Penis name: Coquette

Surprise:
You wouldn't believe the amount of guys who love a chick with a dick. They get it all: girly gorgeousness and a stiff pecker—well, most of the time—wherever they want it.

Confusions:
My penis is the last souvenir of me as a man and I want to keep it because it makes me unique and then there are times when it all seems so weird and I don't know what to do.

Coquette says:
"I never get bored living with you."

Erect size: 5.25 inches

HARRY
Penis name: Decapitated Head of Walt Disney

Cheers:
My penis and I have been best friends for 67 years, and it still does most of its old tricks, just not so often. My wife kisses Walt at least once a day. She finds my pecker very amusing.

Regrets:
I wish I had had more sexual adventures in my youth. I never got all the mileage out of my penis that I should have.

Listen:
"Buy yourself some new underwear, for Christ's sake! Didn't Woolworth's go out of business 20 years ago?"

Erect size: 6.25 inches

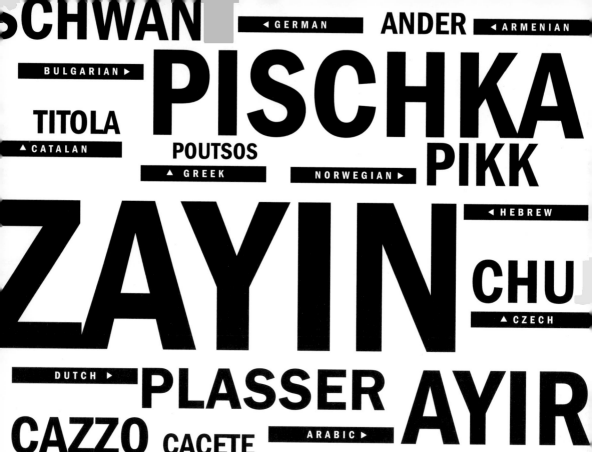

SCHWAN ◄ GERMAN ANDER ◄ ARMENIAN
BULGARIAN ► PISCHKA
TITOLA POUTSOS PIKK
▲ CATALAN ▲ GREEK NORWEGIAN ►
ZAYIN ◄ HEBREW
CHU
▲ CZECH
DUTCH ► PLASSER AYIR
CAZZO CACETE ARABIC ► ORTABACAK
▲ ITALIAN ▲ PORTUGUESE
TITTLINGUR KONTOL ◄ INDONESIAN ▲ TURKISH
▲ ICELANDIC
PULA SWEDISH ► KUK
◄ ROMANIAN

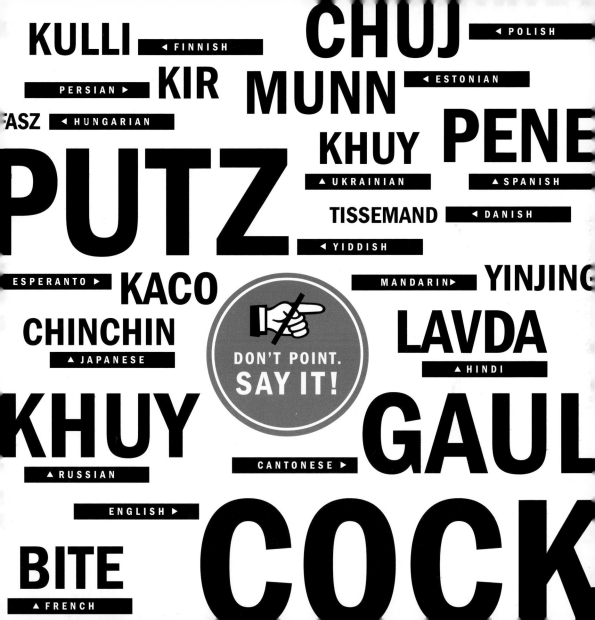

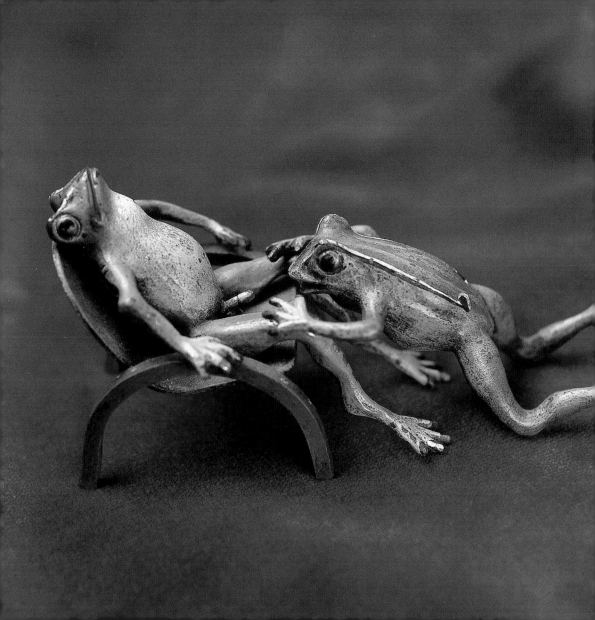

"Hey, hop on over to my pad
and I'll give you a blow job."

Somehow, it sounded more poetic when the ancient Greeks called it "playing the flute." Or when the Kama Sutra's scribes referred to it as *ambarchusi*, "sucking a mango."

Fellatio, from the Latin verb *fellare*, "to suck," has been around forever because it's such a simple and satisfying concept: a mouth on a penis. It can take place in an elevator, for the thrill of a quickie. Or on a satin-covered bed, with both partners pleasuring each other in a slurpy *soixante-neuf* co-mingle. Some men go absolutely wild being oral sexed while sitting buck naked on the kitchen counter. Many love it with their testicles pulled or a finger probing their anal opening. And then there are the Antarctic devotees, who crave the frosty zing of a mouth filled with ice cubes.

Many recipients find it impossible to achieve orgasm during oral sex, no matter how experienced the tongue flicker. No problem. Sucking is just one item on a grand sexual menu. And swallowing a hot load isn't everybody's idea of a fruit smoothie. Or a terrific example of safe sex.

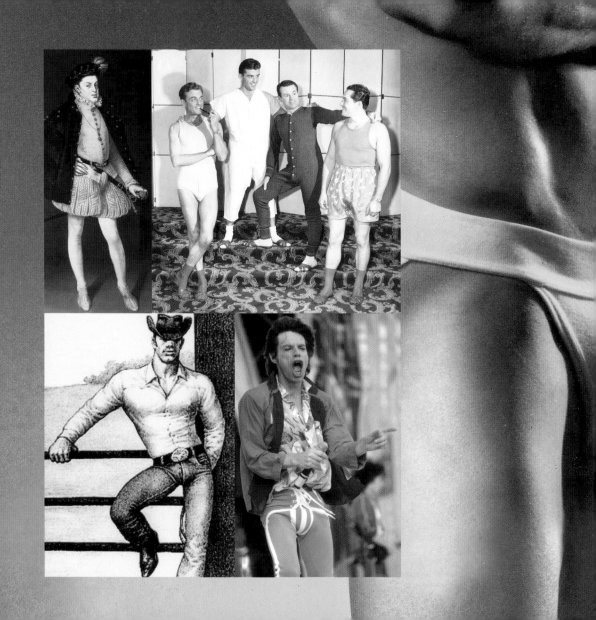

LOVE THAT BULGE!

Nothing like having your jewel-encrusted codpiece enter a room before you do. For royalty, soldiers and uppercrust gents of the 15th-16th centuries, this crotch-aggrandizing protrusion was a symbol of unstoppable virility and peacockian vanity. Codpieces of eye-opening proportions were integrated into suits of armor to shrivel the enemy. When things quieted down, codpieces doubled as pockets for change. Legend even has it that Henry VIII stuffed his ample braguette with medicine-soaked bandages to quell his raging syphilis.

Happy and healthy, the bulge remains a mound of delight. Released from the sexless stupor of underwear pix from vintage Sears catalogues (where peckers were muffled by a slice of white bread tucked inside the front pouch), the manly package gets rock 'n' roll sweaty and totally Jagger-licious. Tom of Finland pumps up the basket and defies the limits of the buttoned fly. Calvin testosterones Times Square with his hunky billboards. And Australian lifeguards make us fantasize about drowning down under. Beautiful bulges. Everywhere. Set your eyes into 4-wheel drive and follow the curves.

PAINT YOUR
WALLS

Ivory Tower

Cockeyed
Curry

Manly
Mahogany

Mocha
Cream

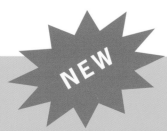

NEW

DELUXE FAUX FINISHES

Trickier...but worth it!

TO MATCH YOUR
PENIS

Prickly Pink

Raging Red

Honey Pie

Pouting Purple

Pubissimo

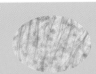

Frecklehead

You're So Vein

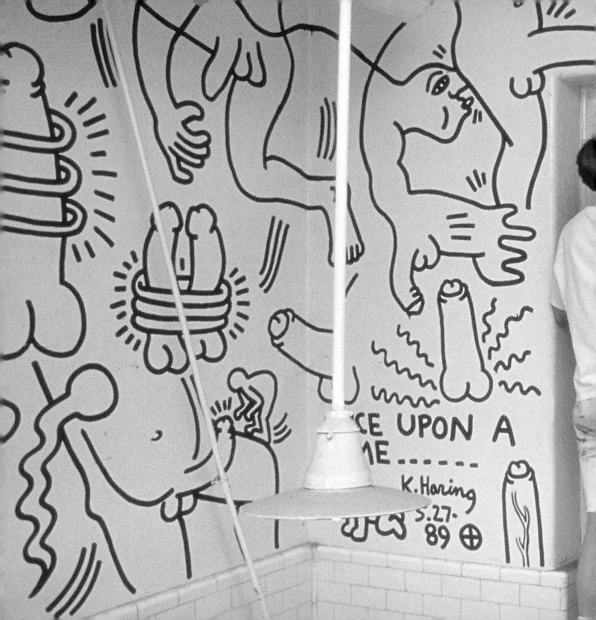

CE UPON A
ME.......

K. Haring
5.27.
89 ⊕

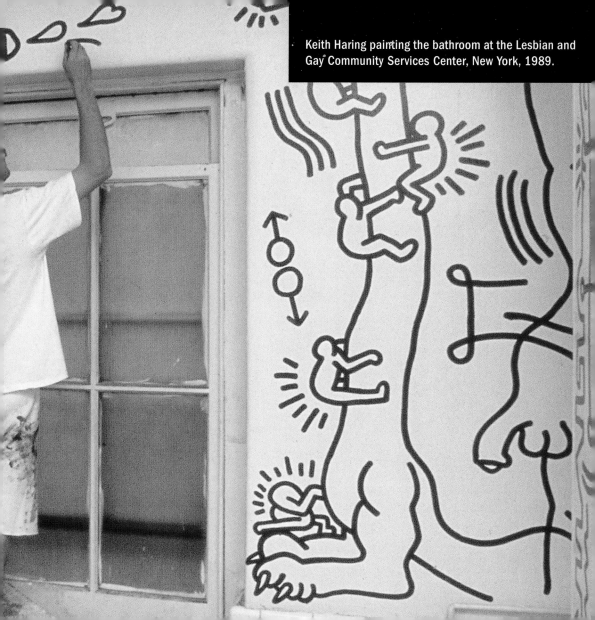

Keith Haring painting the bathroom at the Lesbian and Gay Community Services Center, New York, 1989.

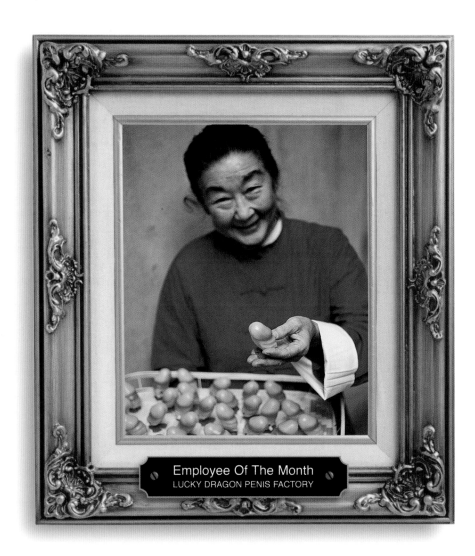

Employee Of The Month
LUCKY DRAGON PENIS FACTORY

"All day long make penis hop...make penis hop. Sometime foot fall off...spring pop and hit me in eye. More quick...make more happy penis boss say. Three hundred I make today...not enough...make more. May Wong at table next say her penis hop the biggest. You look like penis I say. She angry...later she laugh and laugh. I do job...go home and make egg drop soup for husband. No see his penis for three years."

—CHING LEE

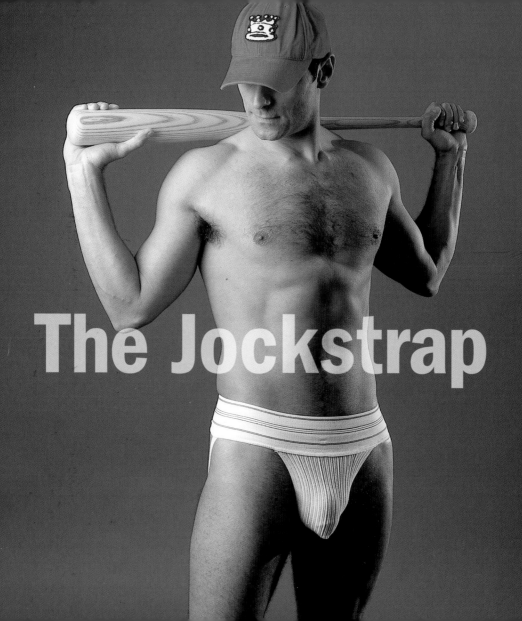

The Jockstrap

The average male will own six jockstraps from ages 12 to 60.

Jockstraps have been around since 1874. The Bike Web Manufacturing Company engineered an athletic supporter to provide relief for bicycle jockeys tortured by the cobblestone streets of Boston. The "bike jockey strap" soon became known as the "jock strap." And the business of genital protection was off and running.

Remember the embarrassment of asking dad to buy your first jockstrap for gym class. "Gotta protect those testicles, son" came a fatherly reply as he handed over a contraption that would add its tantalizing bouquet to your locker for the rest of the year.

Good news, gals. Savvy manufacturers are now featuring female protective cups designed to prevent injuries to *your* pelvic region. Current color: white. Victoria's Secret, take note.

Into used jockstraps? You're not alone. The Web (search: athletic supporters) is filled with eclectic recyclers who like 'em with a sweaty pedigree.

Testicles pack the greatest concentration of nerves in the male body. The smartest athlete sports a hard protective cup inside his jock...or takes a softer approach with a flexible cup or compression performance shorts. The biggest challenge: getting school-age players to wear something more protective than ball-jangling boxer shorts.

"And now he's tiny, and soft like a little bud of life!"

D.H. Lawrence, *Lady Chatterly's Lover*

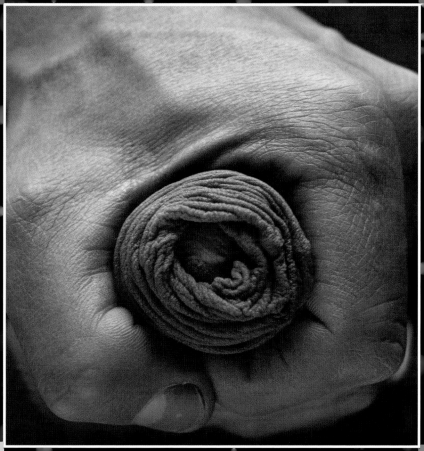

THE GREAT CIRCUMCISION DEBATE

TWENTY-FIVE YEARS AGO, ALMOST 90 PERCENT OF AMERICA'S NEWBORN BOYS SAID FAREWELL TO FORESKINS THEY BARELY KNEW. TODAY, THAT SNIP, SNIP INTO MANHOOD IS ANYTHING BUT STANDARD PROCEDURE. FORESKINS ARE BACK IN A BIG WAY. ARGUMENTS PRO AND CON ARE PASSIONATE. TURTLENECK OR NOT, YOU DECIDE.

Let's hear it for tradition. If it was good enough for King David, Kirk Douglas and Prince Charles (who was attended to by London's premier *mohel*), why rock the boat? Advocates of circumcision cite a well-documented list of health benefits. For starters, circumcised infants are much less susceptible to urinary tract infection. The procedure virtually precludes penile cancer and eliminates balanoposthitis (an inflammation of the foreskin and glans usually caused by poor hygiene). Studies also reveal that circumcised men are at least twice as unlikely to catch herpes, syphilis and HIV during unsafe sex. And millions of folks just love that exposed "mushroom" head.

Anti-circumcision advocates are hardly sitting silently in the corner. They consider the procedure an inhumane act of genital mutilation (frequently performed without anesthesia), encoding the developing brain with pain instead of pleasure. Improved hygiene standards, they argue, have made foreskin-related diseases and infections increasingly rare. Advocates for intact penises assert that the numerous nerve endings in the foreskin and its gliding action contribute greatly to a man's sexual pleasure. It protects and lubricates the glans, which, with circumcision, often becomes less sensitive over the years. Their bottom line: Why would anyone want to discard the best part?

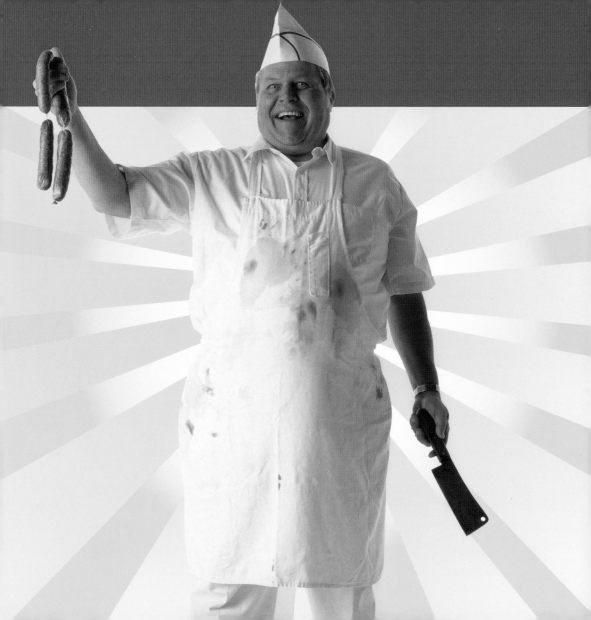

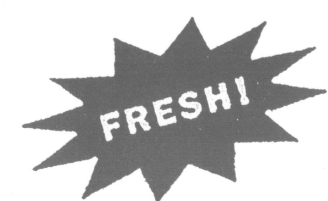

FRESH!

Foreskins for **Sale**

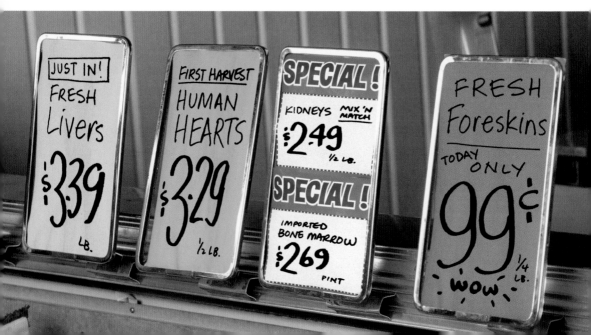

JUST IN!
FRESH
Livers
$3.39
LB.

FIRST HARVEST
HUMAN
HEARTS
$3.29
½ LB.

SPECIAL!
KIDNEYS MIX 'N MATCH
$2.49
½ LB.

SPECIAL!
IMPORTED BONE MARROW
$2.69
PINT

FRESH
Foreskins
TODAY ONLY
99¢
WOW
¼ LB.

Ever wonder what hospitals do with a baby's foreskin once it's been removed? More often than not, this precious calamari isn't headed for the trash can.

Over the past two decades, hundreds of thousands of discarded foreskins have been sold to pharmaceutical companies and bio-research laboratories, which require young skin cells for clinical investigation and for the burgeoning field of artificial skin technology. One stamp-sized piece of foreskin contains enough genetic material to grow 200,000 units of faux skin.

For many, the promise of laboratory-created skin with living human epidermal and dermal cells is extraordinary, opening up major new avenues for the treatment of burns and wounds. For those who view circumcision as barbaric, the business of "harvesting" foreskins is an even greater insult. They ask: Who is the legal owner of a baby's foreskin after it has been cut off? And is it ethical for a hospital to sell a baby's foreskin without telling his parents—and keep the money?

…eeth, *v.t.* to smooth. [....]

smeg′mȧ, *n.* [Gr. *smēgma*, soap.] in physiology, a thick, cheesy secretion found under the prepuce in males and around the clitoris and labia minora in females.

smeg·mat′iç, *a.* being of the nature of ....

.... smelled or sm....

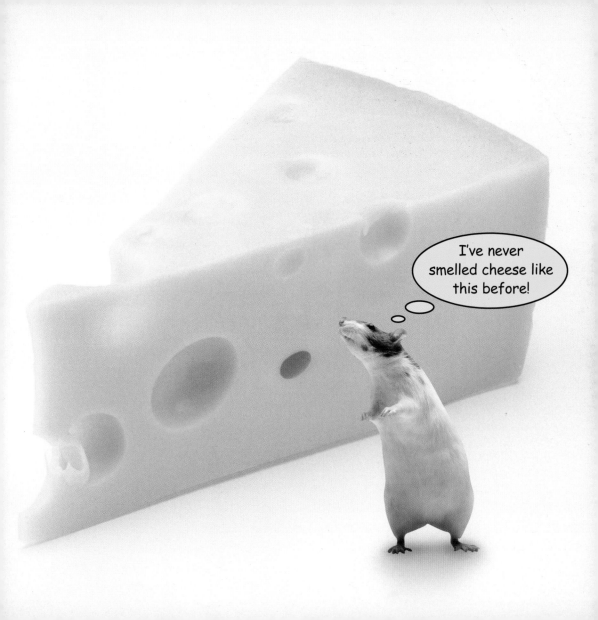

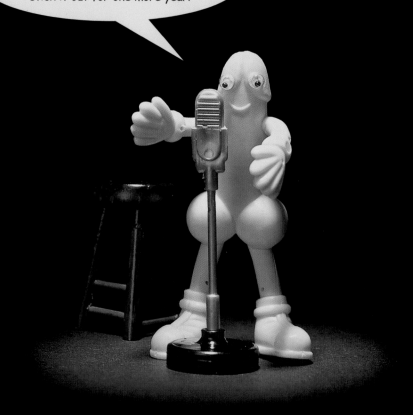

"God gave us a penis and a brain,
but only enough blood to run one at a time."

ROBIN WILLIAMS

If I grew
an inch with
every penis
enlargement
spam...

In just
one year
I'd have
a 43-foot
penis!*

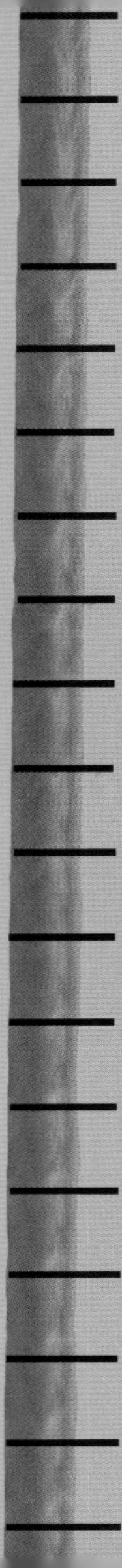

You know what she wants

WANNA BE A BIG BOY?

Two Beautiful Inches Guaranteed!

Everybody loves a BIG PENIS

Forget the rest, this works

Expand your manhood right now

Give your dick a new lease on life

A handful of MANHOOD

Ready for a thicker, longer penis?

The MAGIC penis pill is here!

SIZE really does matter

A whole lot of lovin', thanks to you

Make your tool at least 20% bigger

Salute your flag with a manly penis

THE PROVEN PENIS WONDER ENLARGER

Hey, what's that stuffing your pants?

Nothing is too small for us

The third leg you've always wanted

Grow it. Show it. Here's how!

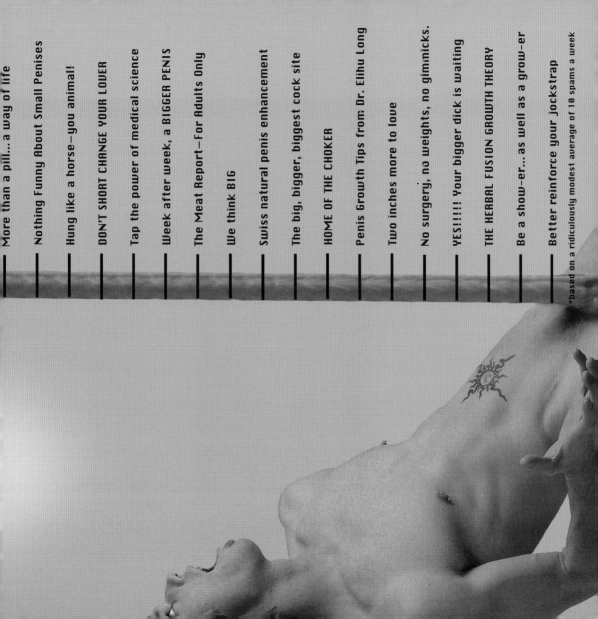

More than a pill...a way of life

Nothing Funny About Small Penises

Hung like a horse—you animal!

DON'T SHORT CHANGE YOUR LOVER

Tap the power of medical science

Week after week, a BIGGER PENIS

The Meat Report—For Adults Only

We think BIG

Swiss natural penis enhancement

The big, bigger, biggest cock site

HOME OF THE CHOKER

Penis Growth Tips from Dr. Elihu Long

Two inches more to love

No surgery, no weights, no gimmicks.

YES!!!!! Your bigger dick is waiting

THE HERBAL FUSION GROWTH THEORY

Be a show-er...as well as a grow-er

Better reinforce your jockstrap

*based on a ridiculously modest average of 10 spams a week

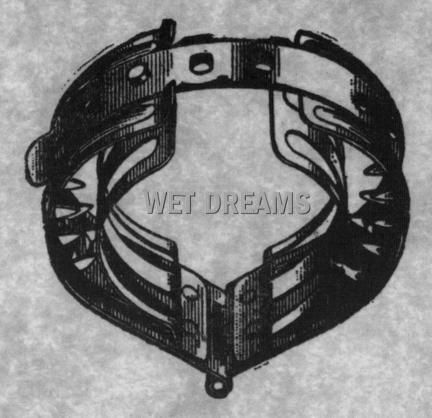

THERE'LL BE NO

WET DREAMS

IN THIS HOUSE!

Somewhere around the age of 13, a boy's sperm factory kicks into high gear. Pumped with testosterone, young lads around the world find their nightly slumbers interrupted by the uncontrollable fireworks of *nocturnal emissions*, better known as wet dreams. Ah, the thrill of ejaculating (it's not uncommon for adolescents to have as many as 10 wet dreams a week). Oh, the confusion of explaining those cardboard-stiff sheets and pajama bottoms to Mom.

In these so-called enlightened times, wet dreams and frequent masturbation urges are considered as natural a rite of passage as pimples and pubic hair. In the late nineteenth century, however, medical authorities in the United States and Europe decreed that the frequent spilling of semen would cause brains to grow dull and genitals to fall off. "The expenditure of the most vital fluids of the system" would surely bring early death.

These dire warnings gave birth to a brand new industry: the creation of anti-wet dream devices. In the user-friendliest contraptions, an expanding penis would cause an alarm to go off, averting seminal spillage. Pity the lad who went to bed wearing **The Timely Warning**, featured at left, patented in 1905 by Dr. Foote's Sanitary Bureau of New York. When an erection stirred, the menacing aluminum teeth were guaranteed to turn the sweetest dream into a living nightmare.

The **urethra** is Route 66 of the penis world, stretching from the **bladder** to the penile opening. Urine and semen travel on it, but not at the same time.

The **prostate** is a male's G-spot, providing a surprising amount of pleasure when massaged. This chestnut-sized sex gland produces the thin, watery fluid that's a prime ingredient in semen. An enlarged prostate can be a real troublemaker, reducing a man's urine stream to a trickle. To stay clear of this and prostate cancer, a yearly digital rectal exam and PSA blood test are best bets.

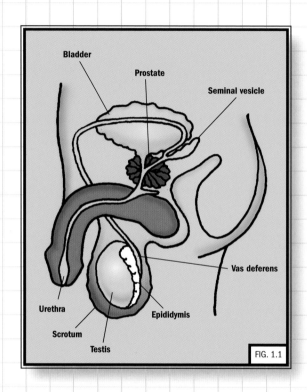

FIG. 1.1

The two **vas deferens** tubes conveying sperm from each testicle to the urethra are also the "vas" in vasectomy. In this common sterilizing procedure, a tiny segment of the tube is severed—end of the road for millions and millions of sperm.

The **epididymis** is a tube-filled mass at the back of the **testicles** where mature sperm enjoy a little siesta before embarking on their expedition up the vas deferens.

Thank you, **corpora cavernosa**. During sexual arousal, these two large spongy cylinders expand considerably as they fill with blood—about 10 times the amount of blood found in a flaccid penis. This hydraulic spectacle continues during sleep, also. Snoozing males usually experience hard-ons every 70 to 100 minutes, and sexy dreams have nothing to do with it. The penis is simply being reinvigorated with fresh oxygen and blood.

p.s.: there are no bones in the proverbial boner.

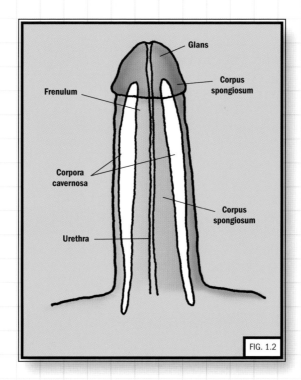

Glans

Corpus spongiosum

Frenulum

Corpora cavernosa

Corpus spongiosum

Urethra

FIG. 1.2

Behold the **glans**, the head of the penis, consisting of soft tissue called **corpus spongiosum**. Glans is Latin for acorn.

Lots more **corpus spongiosum.**

It feels so good. The **frenulum** is a hotbed of sensitivity just below the glans on the underside of the penis.

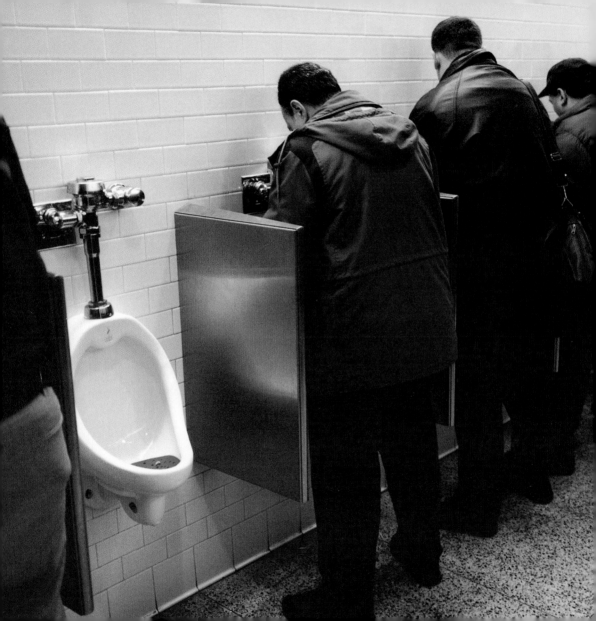

Urinal Etiquette

Refrain from whistling "The Man I Love" while peeing.

Avoid the temptation of saying: "Nice watch you got there."

If you must fart, don't make it a long-winded affair.

On those rare occasions when you have to use the little boy's urinal,
do not get on your knees.

Should you sense the guy next to you is piss shy, never comment:
"It's all in your head."

Be courteous when people are standing behind you.
Shake no more than three times.

Don't hog the hot air dryer trying to dry those last drops
on your pants. Hide your little puddle with a highly regarded
newspaper or a fine cashmere topcoat.

DO IT YOURSELF

The dream goes something like this: You're naked at home, sitting on a chair with a rather sizable erection keeping you company. You bend your head down...and to your amazement, you effortlessly put your mouth over the head of your penis. "Boy, that was pretty easy," you say to yourself. "No big deal. I should do this more often!" And that's why they're called dreams. Unless you were born into a family of double-jointed circus performers from Romania, sucking your own noodle is a tough assignment. But try to find a guy who hasn't tried it.

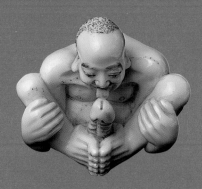

Once, when I was 17, I touched my dick with the tip of my nose. I'm 43 now
and sometimes I get a back spasm wiping my ass.

ALEX, LOUISVILLE

I would love to be able to suck myself off.
It's as queer as you can get without being queer.

ANTHONY, DALLAS

My girlfriend said she would take me to Acapulco if I could blow myself.
I got as far as Coney Island.

JULIO, NEW YORK

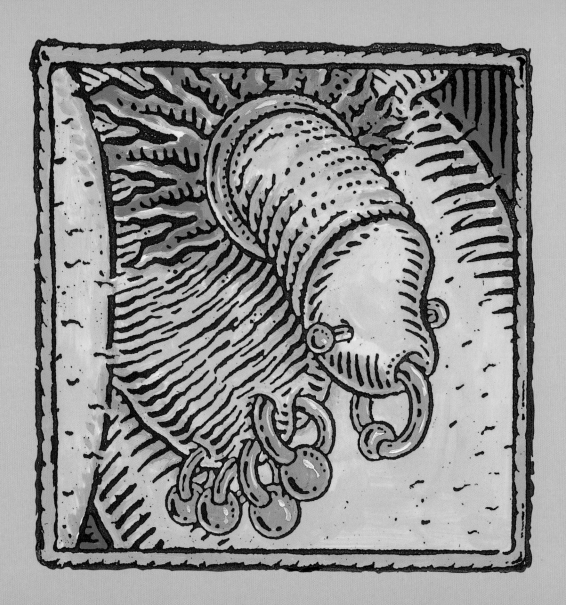

Prince Albert, you kinky devil.

"OUCH!"

It's a natural reaction if you've never seen a pierced penis before. And why would anyone name them after the husband of Queen Victoria?

Documents and diaries reveal that the penile heads of many upper-crust gentlemen during the Victorian era were pierced with a "dressing ring" used to firmly secure the male genitalia in either the left or right pant leg to prevent unsightly bulges. (Aren't you glad you were born a few years later?)

Today, bulges are celebrated and genital piercing is bigger than ever. Converts claim that piercing intensifies every orgasm for the male by stimulating the nerves that end in the glans of the penis. Their female partners rave about their intensified pleasure and heightened orgasms. In fact, there are many women who wouldn't dream of wasting their time with an unpierced wiener.

If you're considering costume jewelry south of the border, better know the lingo. The classic ring piercing the urethra and glans is called a *Prince Albert*. That barbell device through the head is called an *ampallang*, while a variation of this is called an *apadravya*. Add a bunch of flashy *hafadas* on your scrotum, *guiche* rings at the perineum and your favorite *cock rings* to lift and separate...and you're ready for anything. Best of all, there's no need to fret about airport metal detectors. Surgical stainless steel shouldn't cause a bleep on the radar screen.

How much? Genital piercing rates at New York Adorned in Manhattan's East Village average $30 per piercing, with jewelry accessories starting at $40. Fair is fair: Piercings of the inner labia and clitoral hood cost pretty much the same.

Hurt? While most guys reading this page are holding their crotches by now, Prince Alberts really aren't that painful...less of a zap than getting one's nipples pierced.

Peeing suggestions? Careful. Your straight stream of the past will now look like a watering can. Get close to the bowl. And those first few whizzes are sure to be stingers.

fabulous *sleezy* *old-fashioned*

SEX TIPS

Masturbate together

It's the best of going solo, with company spicing up the basic recipe. Mutual wanking has all the right ingredients: exhibitionism, kinkiness, selfishness, moans, minimal performance anxiety. You can be tenderly side-by-side in bed. Or across the room (or country). Check your inhibitions at the front door. And, every now and then, check to see what's really turning on your favorite co-conspirator.

Fantasize: anything goes

Remember that luscious office intern with the Lycra-swathed behind? How about that UPS hunk, kissed with summer sweat in all the right places? And what about that Palm Springs pool porno, where they did the most amazing things with Bain de Soleil? Guys, take 'em all to bed with you! Fantasies are the world's greatest turn-ons. They allow us to have sex with anyone and anything, while keeping us faithful and germ free. Be creative. Be outrageous.

new-age   quick & easy   nice & slow

FOR GUYS

Stick it where the sun don't shine

We know what you're thinking. Well, think again…about the world of slippery toys that never make it to F.A.O. Schwarz. There's something so wonderfully tawdry about sexual accoutrements: vibrating masturbation sleeves and life-size autographed "pussies" of your favorite nymphettes. But why waste those Duracells, when you can plug a succulent honeydew or a hoagie lathered in Hellman's. Friendly advice: avoid vacuum cleaners and hollow tree stumps (you never know what's lurking inside).

Slow down and enjoy the ride

The average *shtup* according to Kinsey barely lasts two minutes. Forget the speed race and take your time. Just before you reach the point of inevitability, stop thrusting and take deep breaths. Tug your balls to help delay orgasm. Or squeeze the tip of your penis. When Vesuvius settles down, start pumping again. Then pause. Train yourself to experience the happy quivers of multiple mini-orgasms without ejaculation. They're a delectable appetizer before the big pop.

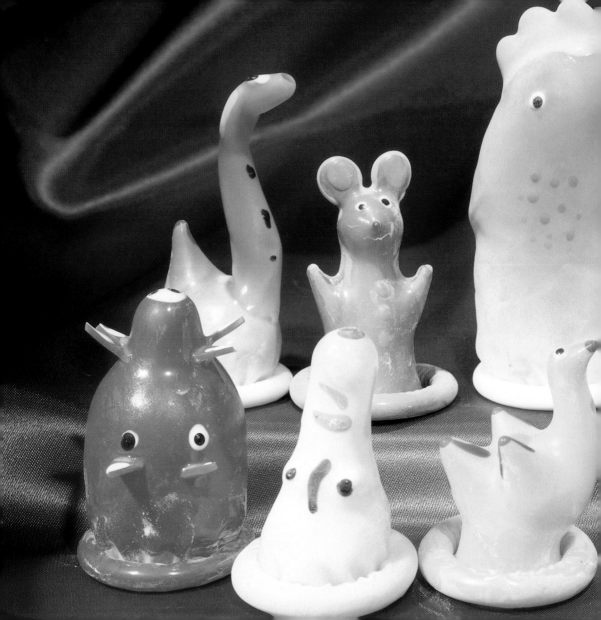

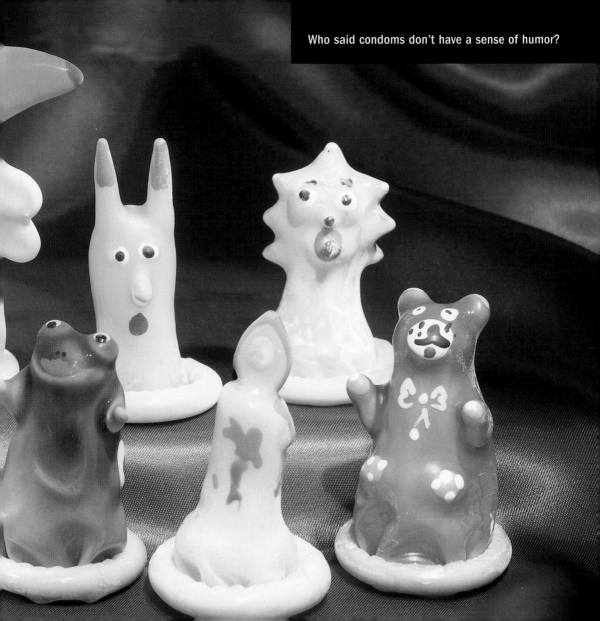

Who said condoms don't have a sense of humor?

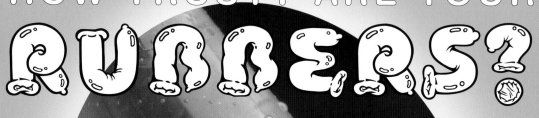

HOW TRUSTY ARE YOUR RUBBERS?

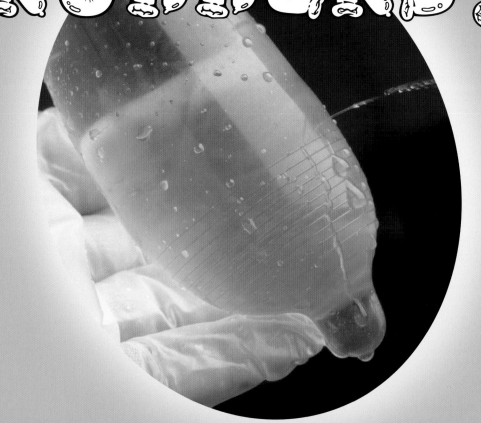

The facts are shocking!

Among prophylactic testers, there's only one mantra: It's got to be perfect or out it goes. (Perhaps the condom industry could have a nice little chat with the automobile industry.) The biggest players in the global condom empire are sticklers for perfection, adhering to the incredibly stringent quality guidelines of the International Standards Organization.

Test #1, The Shocker. Every condom coming off the assembly line is stretched over a metal form, then treated to a high voltage zap. In a split second, any micro weakness in the latex film is discovered and that condom is instantly rejected.

Test #2, The Big Bubble. Part science, part Bazooka. In this test of tensile strength and elasticity, samples from every new batch of condoms are filled with a fixed amount of air until they reach the bursting point. Samples that "pop" too quickly often lead to an entire production run being discarded.

Test #3, The Wet Dream. Condom samples are filled with 300 milliliters of water to test for leakage and suspended for three minutes. Next, they're rolled on blotting paper in search of moisture. Should a few dewy drops appear, chances are excellent that the complete batch will be scrapped.

Test #4, The Old Geezer. In this procedure, samples are artificially aged at high temperatures, so that their efficacy can be tested at the end of their "five year" shelf life. And the codgers that don't make the grade? No retirement home for them, just a visit to the dump.

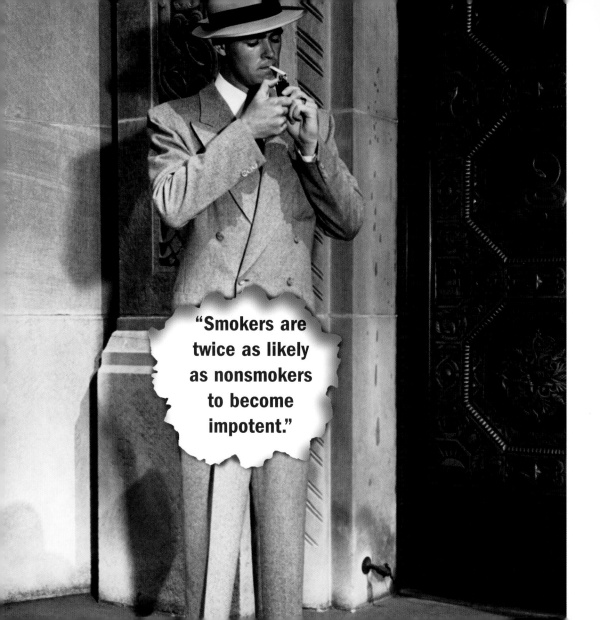

Erections—they're going up in smoke.

We've all seen the classic cliché from Hollywood: a couple lighting up after a fabulous round of lovemaking. It's a rather ironic vignette, when you realize that smoking is one of the leading causes of impotence.

Medical studies confirm that smokers are twice as likely as nonsmokers to experience erectile dysfunction and diminished sex drive...a sobering fact that has yet to join the dire cigarette pack warnings most puffers prefer to ignore. Smoking damages the blood vessels in the penis, inhibiting the healthy flow of blood that leads to an erection. Since these vessels are considerably narrower than those leading to the heart, the penis is even more susceptible to the serious effects of smoking. A limp member is also recognized as an early warning sign that heart disease isn't too many ashtrays away.

Wait. There's a bright note in all this. While most smokers, especially those under age 30, refuse to quit over the potential damage to their hearts and lungs, the fear of giving up a satisfying sex life has seduced a substantial new wave of anti-nicotine converts. You decide: a pack or two a day. Or a lusty roll in the hay.

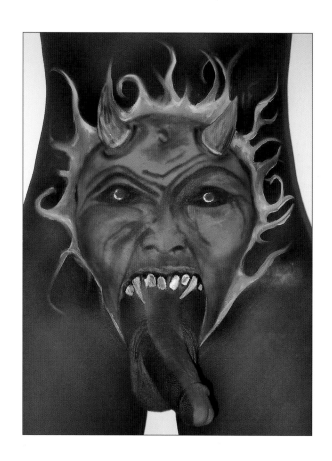

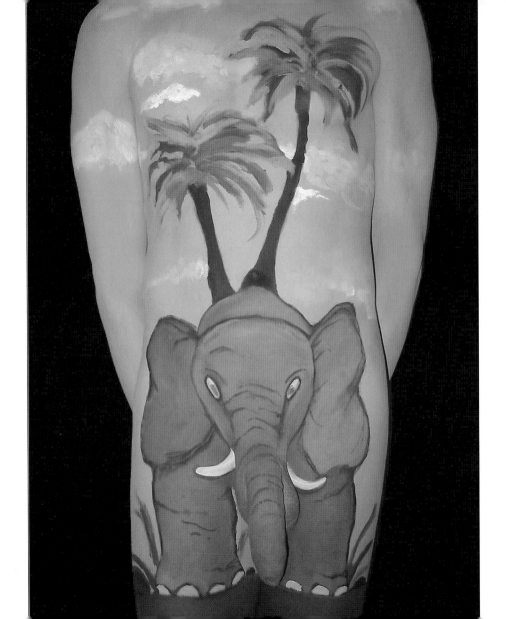

NOODLES
IN THE NEWS

FISHERMEN DIE AFTER FISH BITE OFF PENISES

Two fishermen from Papua, New Guinea bled to death after their penises were bitten off by piranha-like fish in the Sepik River.

As the men were urinating, these ferocious little fish immediately detected a chemical change in the water and swam up the warm yellow stream, deftly biting off the Papuans' *ikibikis* with their razor sharp teeth.

★ ★ ★
SCHOOL BUS DRIVER GOES PENIS SLAPHAPPY

A Montana school bus driver has been charged with assault for slapping a 12-year-old passenger who kept on shouting "penis" at the top of his lungs. The boy insisted it was a scientific term and not a derogatory word. Meanwhile, a more unflappable driver has taken over the route.

★ ★ ★

★ ★ ★
FREQUENT MASTURBATION MAY WARD OFF PROSTATE CANCER

A recent study of more than 2,000 men in Melbourne, Australia concludes that dudes who ejaculate frequently between the ages of 20 and 40 are less likely to develop prostate cancer down the road. Insatiable, youthful seed-spillers appear to have about a third less prostate cancer risk in later years than fellows who held onto their creamy reserve. Researchers propose that frequent ejaculation prevents semen from building up in the prostate gland, where it runs the risk of becoming carcinogenic. To paraphrase the lead researcher: "Flush those ducts, it's good for you!"

★ ★ ★
ICELANDIC PHALLOLOGICAL MUSEUM PREPARES FOR HUMAN WIENER

Located in happening downtown Reykjavik, this living-room-size museum proudly displays about 180 penises from 70 species of animals. Shriveled members from dolphins, Arctic fox, black rats and beluga whales pickled in formaldehyde, plumped with silicon or stuffed and mounted like trophy plaques will all pale once the most coveted specimen arrives: the preserved penis of *homo sapiens*, a promised donation from a generous chap who, unfortunately, is still very much alive and well.

★ ★ ★

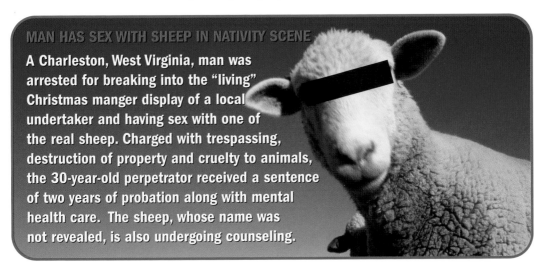

MAN HAS SEX WITH SHEEP IN NATIVITY SCENE

A Charleston, West Virginia, man was arrested for breaking into the "living" Christmas manger display of a local undertaker and having sex with one of the real sheep. Charged with trespassing, destruction of property and cruelty to animals, the 30-year-old perpetrator received a sentence of two years of probation along with mental health care. The sheep, whose name was not revealed, is also undergoing counseling.

71

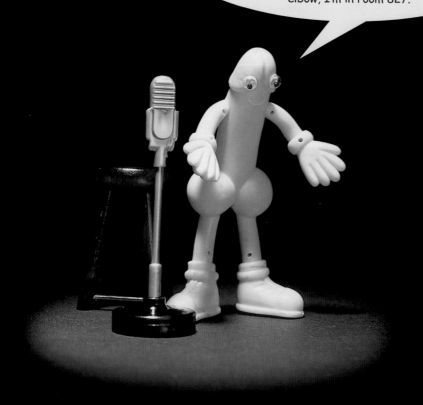

"At my age, I'm envious of a stiff wind."

RODNEY DANGERFIELD

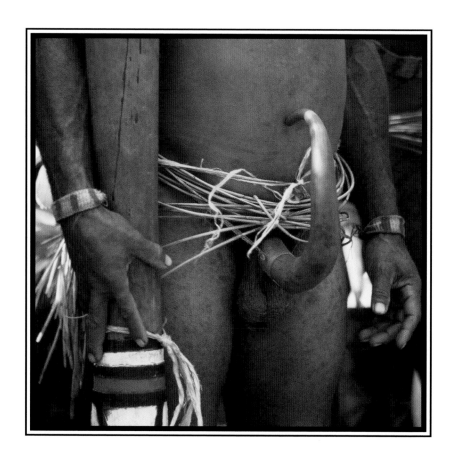

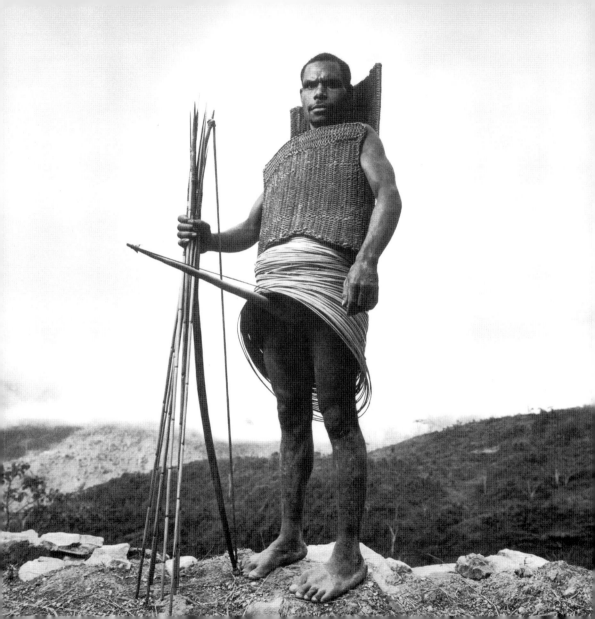

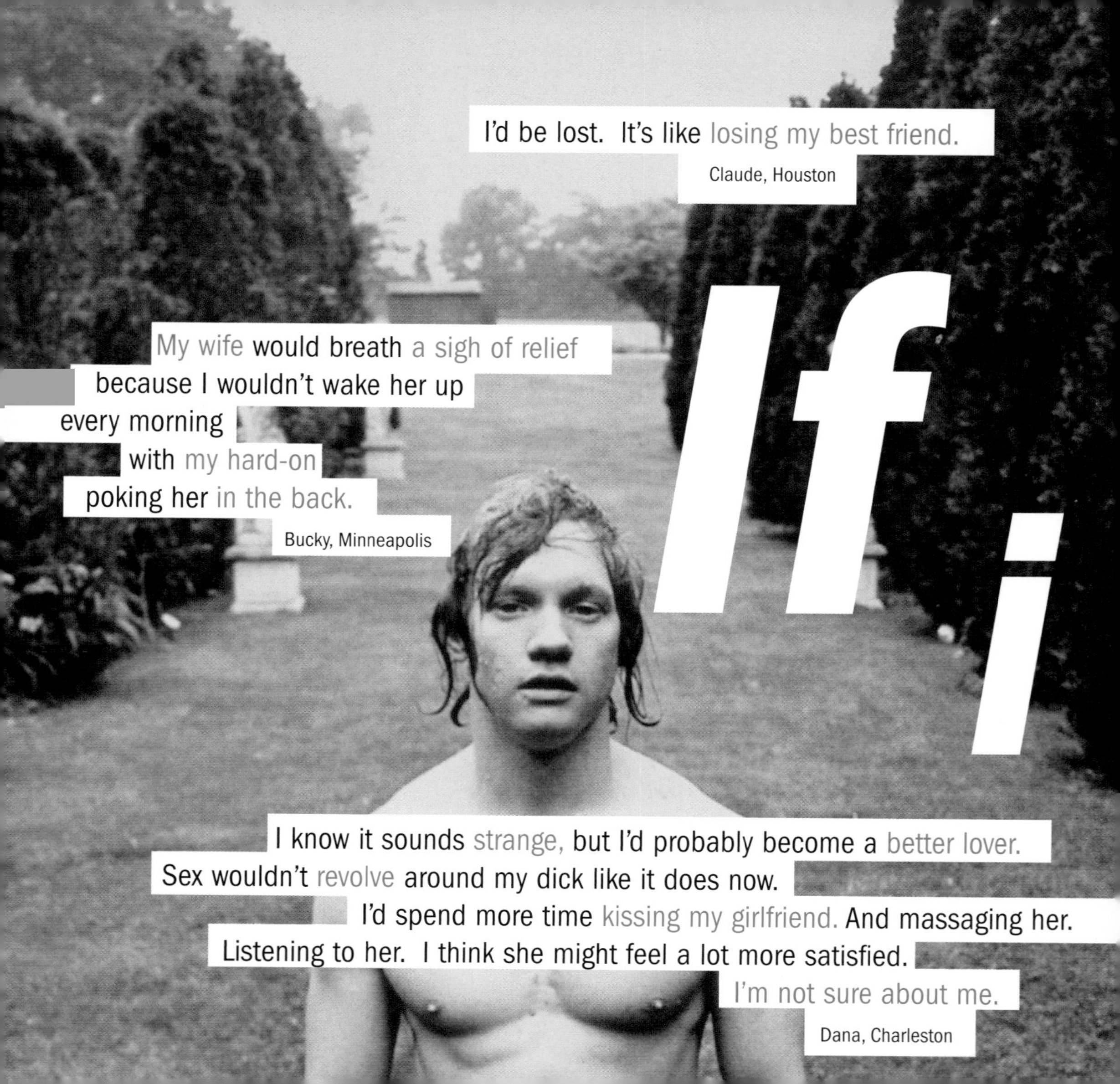

If

I'd be lost. It's like losing my best friend.

Claude, Houston

My wife would breath a sigh of relief because I wouldn't wake her up every morning with my hard-on poking her in the back.

Bucky, Minneapolis

I know it sounds strange, but I'd probably become a better lover. Sex wouldn't revolve around my dick like it does now. I'd spend more time kissing my girlfriend. And massaging her. Listening to her. I think she might feel a lot more satisfied. I'm not sure about me.

Dana, Charleston

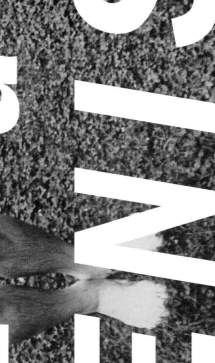

didn't HAVE a PENIS

What would I scratch?

Billy, Kenosha

I don't think I'd be as successful as I am today. Look, here's the way I see it: peckers and balls and testosterone and money are all linked together. No dick, no corner office. Does that make any sense?

Tom, Miami

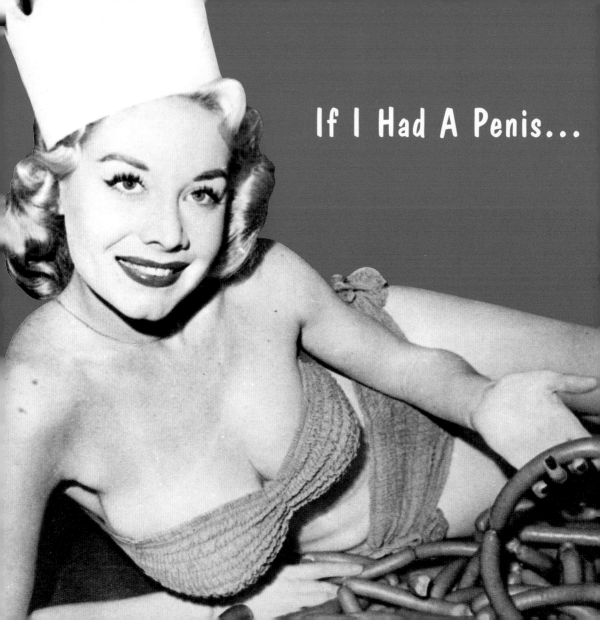
If I Had A Penis...

I'd go hiking a lot, so I could take a leak behind trees whenever I pleased. I'd pee in alleys and fill up an empty Dunkin' Donut cup in my car. I guess it's all about peeing.

RUTH,
NEW YORK CITY

I'd walk down a busy street and have a great time "adjusting" my new bundle in front of everybody. A real turn-on would be standing in front of the mirror and watching my penis...I mean, my cock...get hard.

FRANÇOISE,
BARCELONA

I'd get Prada to design a gorgeous leather jockstrap for me.

LINDA,
WESTPORT

I'd follow my supervisor into the men's room and whip it out at the urinal right next to him. I'd talk about guy stuff. Then I'd shake and zip and head back to my office like it was the most normal thing in the world.

RONI,
SAN FRANCISCO

I would have sex with a beautiful woman as soon as possible, so I'd know what it feels like on the "other side." It would be interesting to discover whether I was an ass "man" or was more excited by a woman's breasts.

SUZY,
CHICAGO

Jesus, I'm confused enough already without one of *those!*

LYNNE,
SANTA FE

I love the idea of donating my seed to a sperm bank...but I'd always wonder if a part of me was out there somewhere.

JEANETTE,
TUCSON

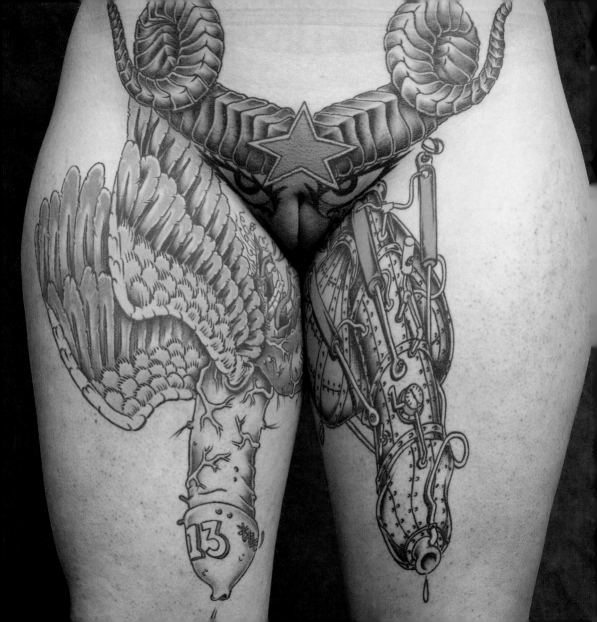

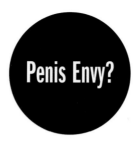

Penis Envy?

Sigmund Freud would be in his glory if this lady knocked on his Vienna door. By the early 1900s, the founder of psychoanalysis was convinced that little girls would reject their own genitals the moment they saw their father's or brother's penis. Girls, Freud expounded, were extremely envious of the male member, believing that their own penises had been castrated by their mothers. Searching for her long-lost penis, a girl would ultimately attach herself to her father. Later, she might find some comfort in the intact penises of other men in her life.

Naturally, the all-male medical community of the time bought this Freudian folly hook, line and sinker. These days, if there's any penis envy still flourishing, it surely exists among men. Straight and gay. Guys are always checking out other guys in the locker room. "Jesus, look at the donkey dong on that little wimp!" And look at those hunks on the screen...in and out, in and out like the hydraulic pumps on the Queen Mary. "Dear God, just another inch or two. Please."

Do women prefer BIG DICKS?

Sure, plenty get totally turned on by size...a real-life "fill 'er up" fantasy. But the majority of women prefer the comfort of an average sized penis *and* a sensitive lover who knows what to do with it. Since most of a woman's sexual pleasure comes from her clitoris and the outer two inches of her vagina (which contain most of the nerve endings), it's a thicker penis that ultimately has a lot more going for it.

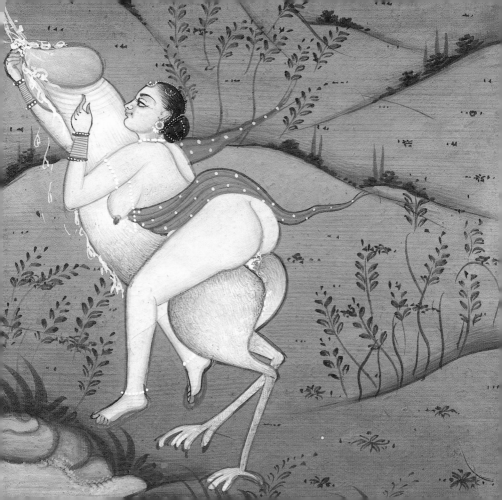

More Oysters For Casanova

"I have loved women to a frenzy" wrote Giacomo Casanova (1725-1798) in his 12-volume memoirs, *History of My Life*. He was a soldier, magician, gambler, spy, a translator of the *Iliad*. But it is Casanova the tireless seducer who reigns supreme, crisscrossing the capitals of Europe in seach of fortune and lust...and the plumpest, freshest oysters that money could buy.

Oysters are the sea's legendary aphrodisiac. Casanova is reported to have consumed 50 of them every morning in the bath, accompanied by the damsel he fancied at the moment. Was it an oyster's vulva-on-the-half-shell imagery that stirred his loins? Or did he know that oysters are abundantly rich in zinc, a key ingredient in the production of sperm and testosterone?

"...we amused ourselves eating oysters, exchanging them when we already had them in our mouths. She gave me hers on her tongue, while I brought mine to her lips; there is no more luscious or voluptuous game between two lovers..."

Giacomo Casanova, *History of My Life*

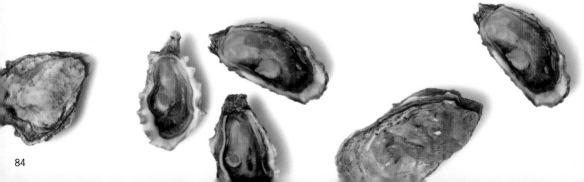

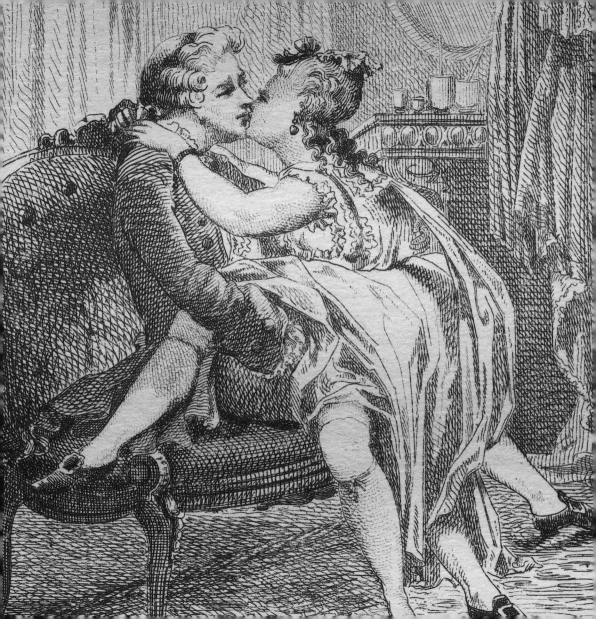

A FABULOUS HOME-COOKED MEAL
(WITH YOU FOR DESSERT)

YOUR LOVER SHAMPOOING YOUR HAIR

A QUICKIE IN AN ELEVATOR

A SLAP ACROSS THE ASS

GUARANTEED TURN-ONS

DIRTY TALK DURING SEX

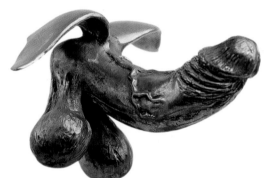

GETTING YOUR ARMPITS LICKED

A PERFECT SMILE

THE DELICIOUS MIX OF PERFUME AND SWEAT

HAVING YOUR UNDERWEAR RIPPED OFF

THREE-WAY SEX FOR THE FIRST TIME

A 90-MINUTE OUTDOOR MASSAGE

THE THRILL OF AN AFFAIR

MAKING LOVE IN A HAMMOCK

LETTING THE NEIGHBORS WATCH YOU
IN ACTION

THE LUXURIOUS EMBRACE OF LINEN SHEETS

A LUSTY PROPOSAL WHISPERED IN YOUR EAR

MAKING LOVE BY A BLAZING FIRE

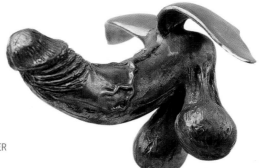

MOANS AND MORE MOANS

A WANDERING TOE

UNDRESSING YOUR LOVER
VERY, VERY SLOWLY

THE SOUND OF A WAILING SAXOPHONE

MAKING LOVE IN THE DUNES

A KISS THAT NEVER ENDS

A BAGFUL OF NAUGHTY TOYS

THOSE WILD AND CRAZY GREEKS

Think Wedgwood and Tupperware with a XXX rating, and you'll understand why some of the friskiest vases and urns from ancient Greece are just emerging from the back rooms of the world's great museums.

The phallus was the very symbol of life and the heart of Greece's decorative arts. The ideal penis was uncircumcised. And surprisingly small…a sure indicator of fertility, according to Aristotle, because the seminal seed had less distance to travel on its way to the uterus.

As you might imagine, the Greeks had grand phallic panoramas for every sexual appetite. Vases are adorned with supple young athletes, their foreskins pulled over the glans and tied with a leather string. (A practice called infibulation, in case you're interested.) Satyrs with huge erections can be observed chasing after prostitutes. Lonely wives are test-driving the newest dildos from Miletus, the dildo capital of the Hellenic age. Group orgies twist around spouts and handles. And platters sizzle with married men caressing their young male lovers.

The facts of life. For the ancient Greeks, they were as close as the china cabinet.

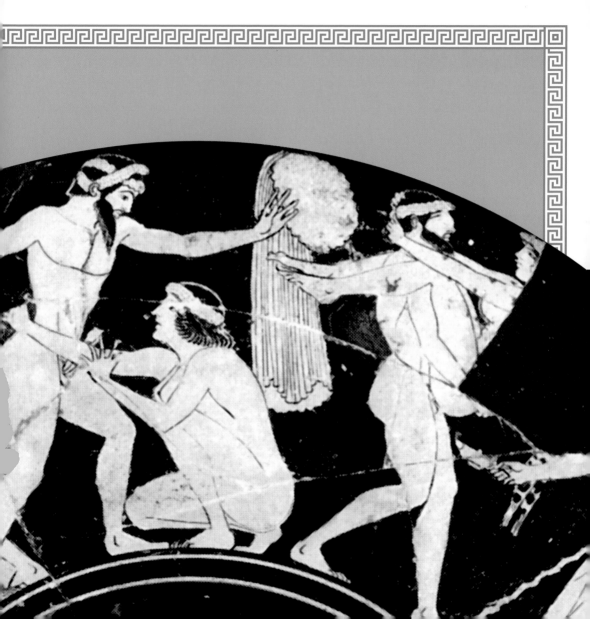

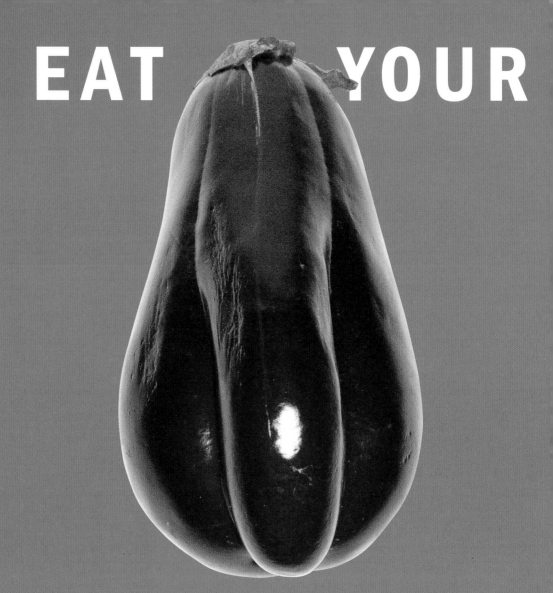

EAT YOUR

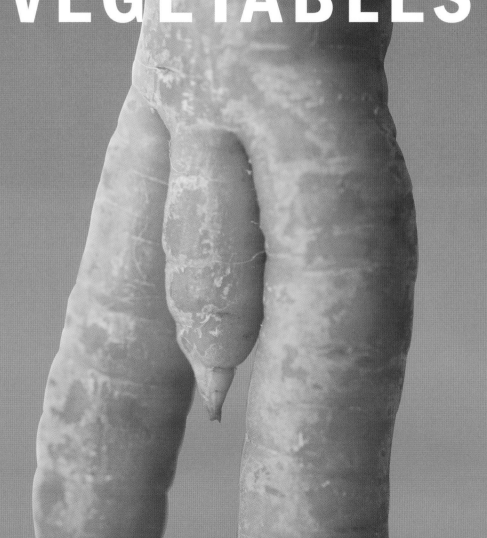

VEGETABLES

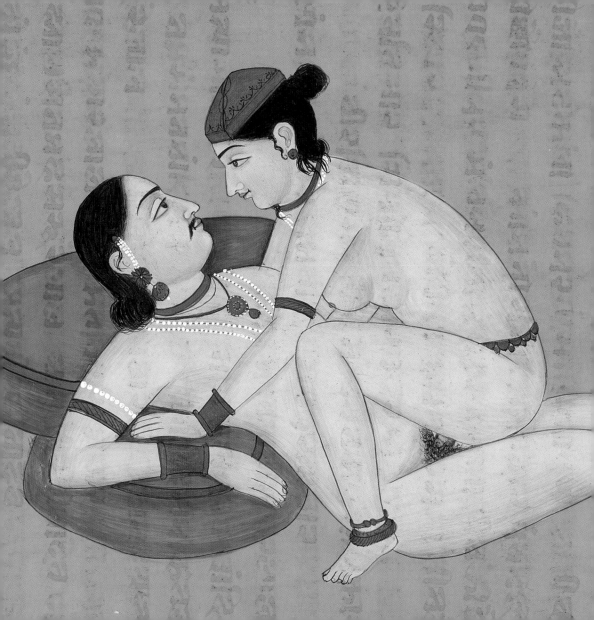

"Then Bahloul inserted his member into the vagina of the Sultan's daughter, and she, settling down upon his engine, allowed it to penetrate entirely into her furnace till nothing more could be seen of it, not the slightest trace...She then gave herself up to an up-and-down dance, moving her bottom like a riddle; to the right and left, and forward and backward; never was there such a dance as this."

Sir Richard F. Burton's translation of *Perfumed Garden of Sheik Nefzaoui*

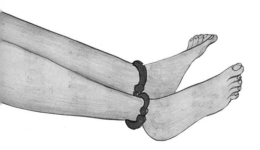

There's a lot more to Japan

than karaoki bars, Louis Vuitton boutiques

and bustling Toyota assembly lines. There's

also a world of eye-opening tradition.

HOUNEN MATSURI

E ach year on March 15, residents of tiny Komaki, about
250 miles south of Tokyo, celebrate a unique fertility festival called
Hounen Matsuri. The mile-long processional route to the shinto shrine of Tagata
Jinja echoes with the sounds of bamboo flutes, saki-satisfied onlookers and the
"hoh-sho hoh-sho" chant of men carrying a giant erect penis. The mighty specimen
shown here was carved from a single cypress tree trunk
by a 90-year-old man. A woody, in every sense of the
word, this 900 pound mega-phallus will be offered at
the shrine as a symbolic prayer for *hounen*, a fruitful year
of abundant harvests and growth for all living things.

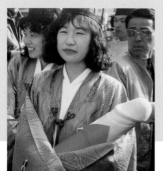

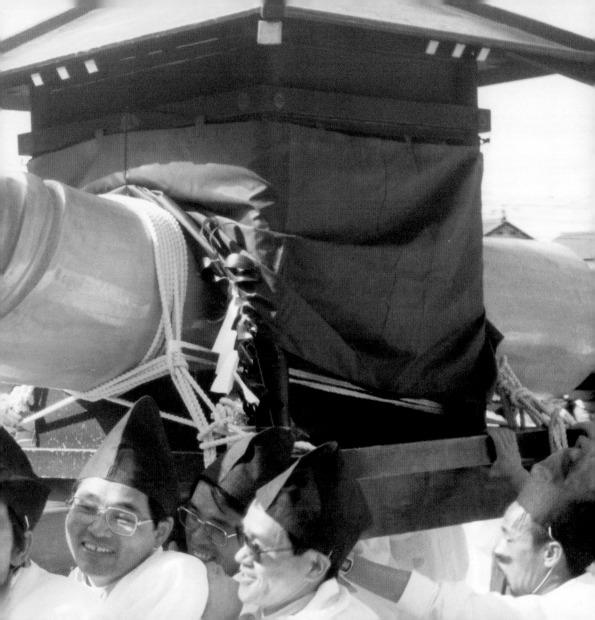

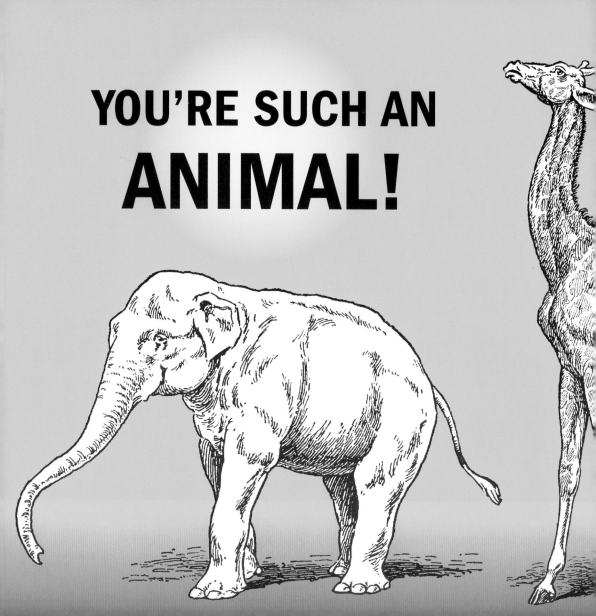

Gorillas may top the scales at 600 pounds, but their erect penises bottom out at around two inches. They don't get to use them much, maybe once a year, since females are in heat only a few days every four years.

Whales sport mega penises of nine feet, making them the real sharks of the deep. They mate once a year, keeping their hoses tucked inside their abdomens between performances.

Pigs' genitals are nature's corkscrews, with a twist that spirals up to 18 inches. This is what we call screwing...no sow ever has to ask, "Are you in yet?"

If your erection was four feet long and 100 pounds, you'd drag it on the ground, too. An **elephant's** penis has a built-in thrusting mechanism, so its owner can gracefully balance his forelegs on his ladyfriend's backside while his pecker does the work. Sex takes less than a minute. Gestation lasts 22 months.

Rising 19 feet and sporting a 24-inch erection, the male **giraffe** knows how to stand out in a crowd. After he shoots his load, he's off with his buddies, having nothing to do with his paramour du jour or her future offspring.

Talk about independence. An **octopus's** penis resides on one of his eight tentacles. When it's time to mate, the entire penis arm detaches and tracks down a female. After copulation, the penis dies, but remains attached to the female.

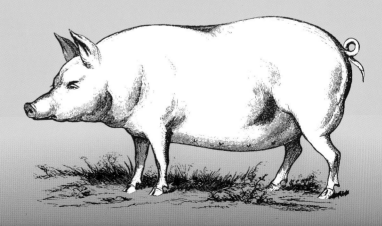

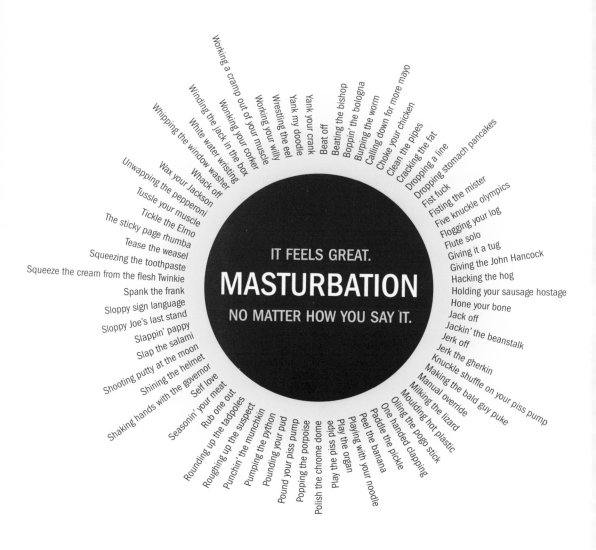

Working a cramp out of your muscle
Working your corker
Winding the jack in the box
Winding the window washer
Whipping the window washer
White water wristing
Whack off
Wax your Jackson
Unwapping the pepperoni
Tussle your muscle
Tickle the Elmo
The sticky page rhumba
Tease the weasel
Squeezing the toothpaste
Squeeze the cream from the flesh Twinkie
Spank the frank
Sloppy sign language
Sloppy Joe's last stand
Slappin' pappy
Slap the salami
Shooting putty at the moon
Shining the helmet
Shaking hands with the governor
Self love
Seasonin' your meat
Rub one out
Rounding up the tadpoles
Roughing up the suspect
Punchin' the munchkin
Pumping the python
Pounding your pud
Pound your piss pump
Popping the porpoise
Polish the chrome dome
Play the piss pipe
Play the organ
Playing with your noodle
Peel the banana
Paddle the pickle
One handed clapping
Oiling the pogo stick
Moulding hot plastic
Milking the lizard
Manual override
Making the bald guy puke
Knuckle shuffle on your piss pump
Jerk the gherkin
Jerk off
Jackin' the beanstalk
Jack off
Hone your bone
Holding your sausage hostage
Hacking the hog
Giving the John Hancock
Giving it a tug
Flute solo
Flogging your log
Five knuckle olympics
Fisting the mister
Fist fuck
Dropping stomach pancakes
Dropping a line
Cracking the fat
Clean the pipes
Choke your chicken
Calling down for more mayo
Burping the worm
Boppin' the bologna
Beating the bishop
Beat off
Yank your crank
Yank my doodle
Wrestling the eel
Working your willy
Working your muscle

IT FEELS GREAT.

MASTURBATION

NO MATTER HOW YOU SAY IT.

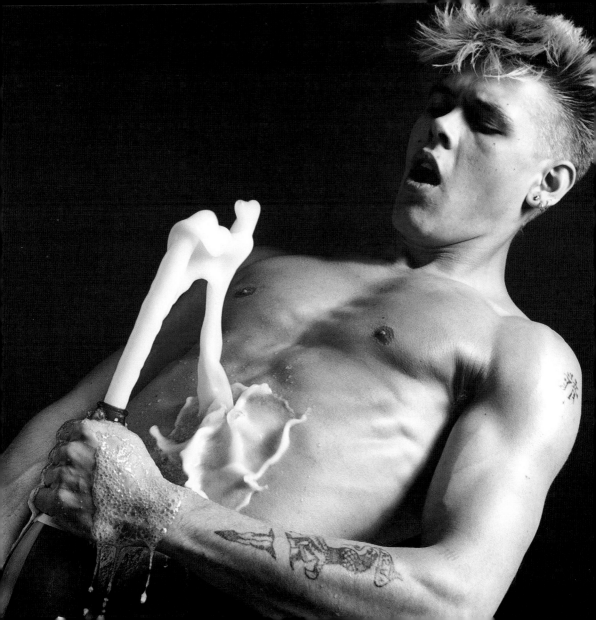

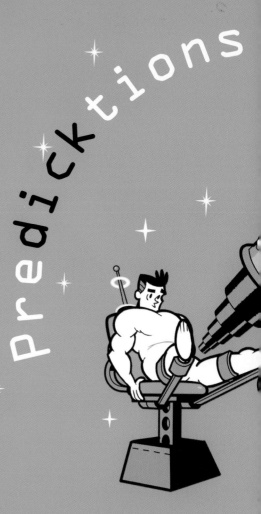

VIRTUAL INTERCOURSE

Blow up dolls are so—what's the word?—tacky. The ultimate joyride will soon be as close as your (extremely) friendly laptop and a fabulous members-only virtual intercourse website. Utilizing 3-D glasses and a revolutionary SensoMatic silicon penis "sleeve," virtual intercourse will offer an almost unlimited range of fantasy encounters and orgasmic opportunities with almost-real babes and boys. Guaranteed to be bug/crab-free.

PENIS ENLARGEMENT... ZAP, ZAP, ZAP

No time to be shy, guy. Spread those legs! Our crystal balls are steaming with excitement, revealing an Inner Glow Laser device that will soon be plumping and lengthening that runty worm of yours without surgery. Don't press us for details...we're only psychics...but a few artfully directed zaps should expand Willy for at least six months.

predicktions

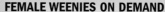

predicktions

FEMALE WEENIES ON DEMAND

Ye olde clit is gettin' ready for the big time. It won't be long before equal-opportunity women sport their own respectable dick-like appendages, thanks to a wondrous capsule that directs a torrent of tissue-expanding blood to the female love button. How big? While clairvoyant images are still a bit hazy, it seems the peckerette will be impressive enough to stop traffic on a nude beach, stir a gin & tonic and freak out an unsuspecting sphincter.

PRIME TIME PECKERS

Lots of adorable flaccid dickeroos are coming to flat screen TVs real soon. And we're talking major network programs, not anything-goes cable. At first, full-frontal treats will sneak their way into comedy shows, in cutesy "Oops,-I-dropped-my-towel" scenes. For more steam and swagger, keep your eyes glued on the afternoon soaps. A promise: your little tykes won't be the only ones drooling.

A PENIS "FACIAL," PLEASE

You heard it here! After years of marinating in ball sweat and pee-pee stains, the penis is about to be Georgette Klinger-fied. First, Dickey and his plums will be lulled to sleep with a warm gauzy wrap steeped in chamomile and lavender. Next, it's time for the fun part: a slippery fruit-whip scruffing massage for the glow of dewy youth. Finally, the pampered rod will be kissed with a rejuvenating mist of concentrated marine proteins. Appropriate tips are still being worked out.

"The good thing about masturbation is that
you don't have to dress up for it."

TRUMAN CAPOTE

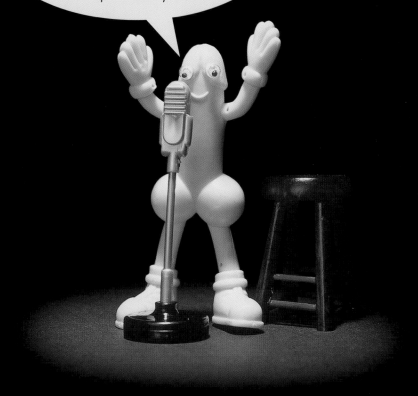

Many believe
the penis was created
for just one purpose.
To bring life
into the world.
Some might disagree.
But who can argue
with the results?

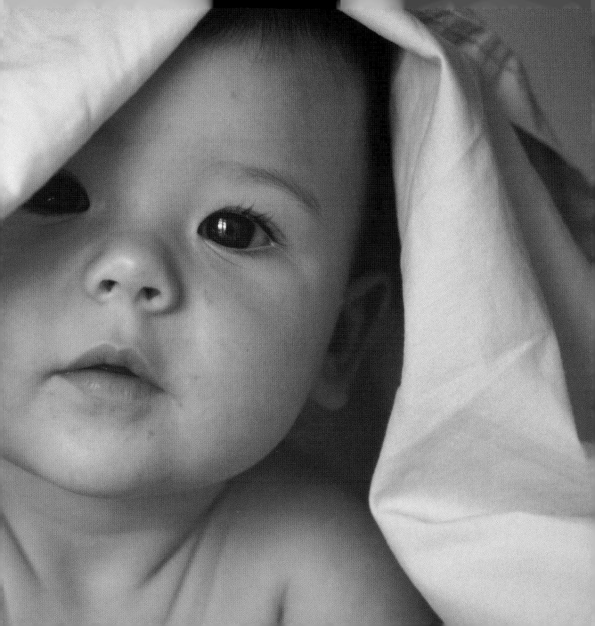

CREDITS

Opposite title page: Lucien Barnes

p. 2: Reed Massengill *Dana Laughing*

pp. 4–5, 6–7, 11, 26, 28 (main photo), 30, 34, 35, 36, 46, 49, 57, 72, 84, 86–87, 103: Studio NYC

pp. 8–9, 13, 41, 42, 45, 51, 66, 71, 104–105: PhotoDisc

p. 14: Sandi Fellman *Taboo*, from her book *The Japanese Tattoo*, Abbeville Press, a source of information for this spread

p. 16: Francesco Urbino *Maiolica Tazza* plate, courtesy of the Ashmolean Museum, Oxford

pp. 18–19: courtesy Pfeizer

pp. 22–23: (except far left photo from SuperStock): Getty Images—all images feature models and are used for illustrative purposes only

Following artwork courtesy Edie Solow of Erotics Gallery, NYC, www.eroticrarities.com: p. 26 (painted Vienna bronze frogs c. 1890), p.57 (contemporary Hong Kong ivory netsuke), p.85 (engraving for *Casanove in Bildern* by Barraud c. 1936), pp. 86–87 (*Winged Phallus* by Doug Johns c. 1980), p. 92 (mid-20th-century Indian painting)

p. 28: (codpiece) The Bridgeman Art Library; (male grouping) Taxi; (Jagger) Hulton Archive; (bottom left illustration) Tom of Finland, detail from *Untitled, 1979*, courtesy of Tom of Finland Foundation, www.tomoffinlandfoundation.org

pp. 32–33: ©1989 Estate of Tseng Kwong Chi and the Estate of Keith Haring

p. 39: ©Carlos Quiroz *Aperture f8*, originally published in Reliquiae, Stéphane Danis publisher, Montreal, 1996

pp. 48–49, generous thanks to Devin Carraway for the inspiration

p. 50: Early 1900s advertising courtesy of Bob McCoy, the Museum of Questionable Medical Devices, www.mtn.org/quack.com

pp. 54, 91: Andreas Sterzing

p. 58: Harvey Redding

pp. 62-63: Nicholas Eveleigh

p. 64: PictureQuest

pp. 68–69: body painting and photographs, Filippo Ioco, www.iocoart.com

p. 70: Taxi

p. 74: CORBIS/Charles & Josette Lenars, Papua, New Guinea

p. 75: CORBIS/Chris Rainier, Highlands of Irian Jaya, Indonesia

pp. 76–77: Arthur Tress *Hermaphrodite*

p. 78: FPG International

p. 80: ©1998 William DeMichele

p. 83: Contemporary Indian painting in the Moghul manner, private collection

pp. 88–89: Athenian plate, 5th century B.C., private collection

p. 90: Frank Degen *Eggplant I*, courtesy Degen-Scharfman, NYC

pp. 94–95: Peter Thoeny, with thanks for the information provided by his web site

p. 99: Irwin Olaf *Joy*, courtesy Wessel O'Connor Gallery

pp. 100–101: Courtesy of Patrick O'Brien/TransFatty.com, illustration by Augenblickstudios.com

THANK YOU SO MUCH

Mom. I'll always remember your asking:
"Why would anyone do a book
about peanuts?"

Bob Simon of Simon Computer Graphics Ltd., NYC.
Bountiful thanks for your creative vision and spirited dedication.
www.simongraphics.com

Edie Solow of Erotics Gallery, NYC.
Art has never been so tempting, or so generously shared.
www.eroticrarities.com

Charlie Conrad. For your enthusiastic thumbs-up
and great ideas.

Jeanette. My fabulous friend
and prickly-pear proofreader.

Toby. Of course.
For always being there.

THE PENIS BOOK
wants you!

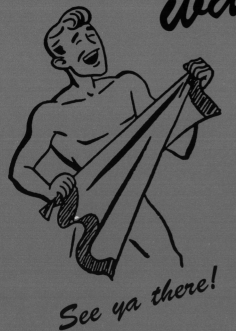

See ya there!

Visit the official website @
www.thepenisbook.com
Here's your chance to tell us
what YOU think about penises
and to learn something
new every time you drop by.